Natural Birth
for the
Mainstream Mama

A practical guide
to achieving a drug-free birth
in a hospital setting

by Lauren Rauseo

Cover and book design by Lauren Rauseo.

Although the author has made every effort to ensure that the information in this book was correct at time of publication, the author does not assume and hereby disclaims any liability to any party for any loss, damage, or disruption caused by errors or omissions, whether such errors or omissions result from negligence, accident, or any other cause.

This book is not intended as a substitute for the medical advice of physicians or medical care providers. The reader should consult a physician or midwife in matters relating to her health and prenatal care.

For Dylan, Liv and Fiona,

who continue to show me that natural birth

was the easiest part of the parenting process

Introduction

"Educate yourself. Know what your options are. If they [medical team] suggest something, know what it means. You can have any sort of birth: a C-section, an epidural, [etc.]. As long as you feel like you are in control, you can have the birth that you want."—Alissa DeBernardo, who used HypnoBirthing as her natural childbirth preparation. After talking with her natural-birthing sister-in-law, she just knew childbirth didn't have to hurt like most people were saying.

Congrats! You are likely expecting a baby and, in opening this book, have just taken an important step in preparing for his or her healthy and peaceful arrival.

Before you take anything I say too seriously, here are my disclaimers.

- I'm not a doctor.
- I'm not a midwife.
- I'm not a labor and delivery nurse.
- I'm not a doula.
- I'm not a childbirth educator.
- I'm not your personal vagina expert.

Maybe one day I'll hold one of those titles (though probably not the one about your vagina), but not today.

So who the heck am I?

I am an ordinary mom, much like you are or are about to be. I create elaborate birthday parties for stuffed animals when my son insists his lovey is turning 4. I use a fish net to get poop out of the bathtub and then throw away all the unfortunate toys that witnessed the incident instead of cleaning them. I mark auspicious occasions like the day my daughter's hair was long enough for pigtails. I love my children dearly, but I sometimes count the hours and minutes until their bedtime when I can go pee by myself.

Like most ordinary people though, I have interests, talents, and passions. My interests are reading historical fiction, running outside with my dog, and taking ridiculously adorable photos of my kids with my fancy camera that I only barely know how to use. My talents are putting words to paper in a way that make them fun to read, and designing websites and printed marketing materials.

My passion is natural childbirth.

While there are facts and statistics in this book (most are even footnoted so you can continue the research on your own), much of what I've written comes from my own opinion and what I've learned during my own journey of becoming a natural birth enthusiast.

While my deepest hope is that you walk away from here feeling empowered for the natural hospital birth that you and your baby wholly deserve, my principal objective in writing this book is to arm moms and moms-to-be with knowledge that may not be provided to them by care providers or by mainstream expectant parent reading. I believe that, as patients, we are in charge of our own health; as mothers, we are in charge of our own paths to a life-changing birth experience. My greatest intention is to leave you more informed than you were before, and itching to learn more. And maybe to make you laugh a little in the process.

Women often say their doctors "delivered" their babies. I don't believe that to be true. We, the mothers, deliver our own babies, regardless of who actually catches them. We do the work. We should also do the research. We must birth our babies ourselves, and so we must become educated about the process ourselves as well.

So with all of that said, sit back with a glass of wine (wait, you're probably pregnant, so scratch that part) and enjoy *Natural Birth for the Mainstream Mama.*

Who should read this book?

This book is the one for you if...

- All of your friends and family members think you're crazy when you bring up the possibility of giving birth without an epidural.
- The idea of birth without drugs intrigues you, but you're a little bit scared to announce your intentions of doing it just in case it's too hard and you don't go through with it.
- Natural birth sounds appealing but you're not sure of all the reasons why it's so good for everyone involved.
- You've heard of home birth and it sounds enticing, but it seems a little too 'out there' for you.
- You like the safety net of a hospital birth setting, but the other stuff that comes with it is turning you off.

This book is NOT for you if...

- You are not totally excited to get personal with your private parts and to hear about what's coming up for you in the next few months.
- You have absolutely zero interest in natural childbirth. I'm not sure why you've gotten this far if that is true for you, but just in case, I wanted to throw that out there. I'm not here to turn you or to tell you that everything you plan to do in birth is wrong. To each her own, and I respect you for making your own informed choices. Rock on.
- You have already read three dozen books on natural childbirth. You're probably all covered. Put the money you were going to pay for this book towards a doula instead.

A few terms to know before you start reading

Obstetrician (OB) – a doctor specializing in obstetrics or the branch of medicine having to do with pregnant women and childbirth. This person went to medical school and is now a competent surgeon. He or she may be an OB/GYN, which means both pregnant women and non-pregnant women are part of his or her practice. In addition to cesarean sections, this doctor can perform other gynecological surgeries.

OBs are experts in pathology, and typically, though not always, follow a medical model of care when handling patients. The main focus is diagnosis and treatment of complications. Interventions are common during labor. The doctors are often decision-makers in the process.

Midwife – a medically trained birth attendant and prenatal caregiver. In the case of a certified nurse midwife (CNM), she would first have been a nurse (usually in Labor & Delivery), and then had additional training (i.e. master's degree) to become a midwife. They are nationally certified by the American College of Nurse Midwives, and are often affiliated with a hospital and doctors for back-up. This person (typically female, though there are a few male midwives) specializes in normal, physiological birth for low-risk women. A midwife is trained to detect issues that arise, but would most likely collaborate with or transfer care to an OB for high-risk cases. Midwives cannot perform surgery, so if a C-section becomes necessary, an OB must step in. However, a CNM can *assist* on C-sections, and co-manage most high-risk pregnancies, especially when they work in groups with physicians.

A certified professional midwife (CPM), unlike a CNM, is typically a direct-entry midwife, which means she was not previously a nurse, and went directly into an accredited midwife training program. CPMs most often work independently and attend births in non-hospital settings. The North American Registry of Midwives is an organization that sets standards for certification of CPMs. And while these midwives are certified, not all states have regulations that license them, and so in some states, the practice of CPMs is illegal.

Midwives are known for using the midwifery model of care for pregnant women. They focus on the health of a pregnancy and view it as a natural process that needs minimal intervention. They view their patients more as equal partners and ultimate decision-makers.[1]

Doula – a non-medical birth attendant who attends to the emotional and physical needs of a laboring woman. Almost always female, this person is there as a constant support person, there throughout labor and birth, solely

---

[1] More on the medical model of care vs. the midwifery model of care:
http://www.ourbodiesourselves.org/book/companion.asp?id=21&compID=121

to comfort and help the mother-to-be and her partner. A doula comple-ments the role the mother's partner plays during labor and birth.

Vaginal birth – baby comes out of vagina.

Cesarean/C-section – baby comes out surgically through an incision in the lower abdomen area.

Natural birth – definition is debatable. More on this in Chapter 1.

Intervention – anything that is introduced during labor or birth that is not physiologically natural. Can include monitoring, medication, surgery, or even coached pushing. Common interventions will be discussed in Chapter 1.

CHAPTER 1

What makes natural birth so freakin' great?

"No matter how you bring your child into this world, it's a life-changing and special time. I'm a huge advocate of natural childbirth because it's something you may not realize you even want to experience until you experience it."—Christie Zimmerman, who says she felt a new and intense respect for her body after giving birth naturally.

Before we can look at why natural birth is so great (and believe me, it truly is), we have to start with what makes un-natural birth not so great. But first, we have to figure out what "natural birth" actually is.

To some people, natural birth simply means vaginal birth or, in other words, not a cesarean section. To others, it means vaginal birth without artificial pain relief.

Still, to others, natural birth means a complete lack of non-natural interventions—this would include all medical pain relief, induction or augmentation (where drugs simulate naturally occurring hormones in order to produce contractions), artificial rupture of membranes (abbreviation is AROM; this means your doctor or care provider breaks your bag of waters), forceps-assisted delivery, vacuum-assisted delivery, the list goes on. It can also include constant electronic fetal monitoring and a saline lock in your vein, even if you don't have anything connected to it. (A saline lock is used often in hospitals for the purpose of keeping a vein open for easy access to administer drugs or other fluids. You could technically wait for it to become necessary to receive said fluids to get it, but in urgent situations, having it already in place can save precious time.)

In this strictest definition, anything that the mother or baby does not control could be seen as an intervention that interrupts the natural physiological process.

If you are giving birth in your home or a birth center (more on these options in Chapter 2), it is certainly possible and even likely that you could achieve that most narrow definition of a natural birth. Many of the interventions mentioned above aren't readily available in those settings, so you'd have to be transferred to a hospital to have them. But in a hospital setting, it is pretty impossible to have your baby with absolutely nothing more than your own sheer will. Even if you wait to come to the hospital until you're fully dilated, you will likely still have time to get a saline lock, which is a common policy at hospitals in the United States.

For me personally, natural birth meant no medical pain relief, and few, if any, other interventions, which I would only accept if I — not just if the care provider — felt were necessary. I readily agreed to the saline lock, as I knew it was hospital policy where I gave birth (and it was used during both of my children's births to deliver fluids and antibiotics to me, and with my second child, Pitocin, as well).

You have to decide what natural birth means to *you*, which elements of that plan you are committed to, and which you are more flexible on. As a pregnant gal, you have probably already heard that not everything goes according to plan, and that you need to be prepared for that possibility. I agree with that sentiment, and can attest to its truth in some way during both of my birth experiences. And while some things really are just dumb luck, it is also true that you have much control over the very things that can lead to everything not going according to plan, so keep reading.

For our purposes, let's assume that "natural birth" means you *definitely want to avoid the following*, except in the case of a true emergency. Don't worry if you don't know what some of these interventions are; I will walk you through each one.

- Cesarean section
- Forceps

- Vacuum
- Episiotomy

And you *strongly want to avoid the following*, but reserve the right to calmly and reasonably consider their use as situations arise:

- Epidural
- Narcotics
- Pitocin
- Constant electronic fetal monitoring
- Artificial rupture of membranes

And you *whole-heartedly believe* in the following:

- Saline lock for IV (this is explained above — it's where the nurse inserts an IV needle and tubing in your arm when you get to the hospital to make it easier to deliver fluids to you, if necessary)
- Intermittent fetal monitoring (this is when your care provider uses either the handheld Doppler every hour or so to listen to your baby's heart, much like they do at all of your prenatal appointments, or an electronic fetal monitor for 15 minutes every hour, where a belt is wrapped around your belly and the baby's heartbeat displays on a screen or a printout next to your bed). The American College of Obstetricians and Gynecologists recommends intermittent monitoring upon arrival to the hospital, and then listening to the fetal heart rate every 30 minutes before, during and after a contraction during active labor. During the pushing phase, the standard is to listen every five minutes.

Okay, now that we have identified what the ideal natural birth might look like, let's talk about why you wouldn't want it any other way.

Why a C-section will surgically ruin your dreams for a natural birth

What is a C-section? Surely you've heard the term and you know that this means the baby comes out through your abdomen instead of your vagina.

C-sections have become so commonplace (even labeled the most common surgery performed in the United States in 2006[2]) that they may not seem like a big deal at all. I have heard people talk about having a C-section with about as much distress as if they were having a pedicure. This is extremely disturbing to me. A C-section is *major surgery*. Like if you were getting your knee replaced or having an organ transplant, except your abdomen is cut open and your internal organs are moved around and exposed. Yeah, not exactly the same laissez-faire attitude you would use for getting a foot massage.

Some women who haven't yet given birth are so scared at the prospect of pushing an 8-pounder out of their hoo-ha, that the idea of a surgical birth actually sounds appealing. Some women who have had C-sections with successful outcomes talk about how much they loved their birth experience — how it was so convenient to know when the baby was coming (in the case of a planned C-section); how it was so fast and completely painless; how they had a long, luxurious stay at the hospital afterwards; how they wouldn't do it any other way. And I'm happy for those women. I'm glad they are pleased with their birth experiences.

And I am so grateful that C-sections are an option for exceptional circumstances when they are necessary.

But for uncomplicated, normal birth — despite the great possibilities that there will be enormous discomfort involved — vaginal birth is just better.

A perfect-case-scenario C-section has the following downsides, all of which don't apply to vaginal birth:

- **Inability to hold your newborn directly after birth.** A nurse or your partner will hold the baby in the vicinity of your head so you can have a peek while your insides are put back inside you and you are closed back up.
- **Delay of breastfeeding** by up to an hour and a half (or longer) until your surgery is complete and until you are physically able to comfortably hold your baby.

---

[2] Study on recent trends in C-sections in the United States:
http://www.cdc.gov/nchs/data/databriefs/db35.pdf

- **Adhesion pain**.
- **Bikini line scar**.
- **Longer hospital stay**. Some women say they enjoy their time at the hospital and speak of it as if they were on a vacation with room service. I didn't have a terrible time at the hospital or anything, but a pool boy interrupting my nap to bring me a fruit kabob is extremely different from a nurse constantly intruding on my time with my baby to lift up a sheet to take a look at my nether regions.
- **Longer recovery once at home**. You have to wait longer to drive, to climb steps, and basically to return to normal functioning life. Taking a forced break sounds good in theory, but post-surgery, you'll want nothing more than to be back to normal and just feel like yourself.

In a not-so-perfect C-section, you are at risk for more serious complications, as well as the aforementioned inconveniences:[3]

- **Infection**, as is a risk with any surgery.
- **Blood loss, blood clot**.
- **Bad reaction to anesthesia** following the surgery, such as nausea, vomiting or headache.
- **Bowel or bladder injuries or issues**.
- **Complications during future pregnancies and future births** (whether those are via repeat C-sections or vaginal births after cesarean, a.k.a. VBACs).
- **Risk for more surgery** to repair something damaged during C-section or possible hysterectomy (not likely but it happens).
- **Death** (extremely rare, but still possible; hey, I'm just telling it like it is).

There are also dangers to your baby when delivered by Cesarean section that are not present for a vaginal birth:

- **A digestive tract that is negatively affected** because he didn't acquire bacteria to colonize the bowel that he would have otherwise

---

[3] More details on risks of C-sections:
http://www.webmd.com/baby/tc/cesarean-section-risks-and-complications

gotten when traveling through the birth canal.[4]

- **Possible increased risk of allergies and asthma**.[5]
- **Accidental premature birth**. Estimated due dates are just estimates. When a baby doesn't choose his own birthday, there is a chance he will be delivered long before he's ready. In the case of a planned C-section at what the doctor believes is 39 weeks, a baby could very well be only 37 weeks' gestation. While a later-term preemie or even a full-term baby at 37 weeks doesn't often have life-threatening or serious problems, he can still experience low birth weight, underdeveloped lungs and robbed time in the womb he could have spent growing. During the final six weeks of pregnancy, a baby's brain doubles in size — that seems like a pretty good reason to stay all up in there if you ask me.[6] It should be noted that in very recent years there has been a major push to delay elective C-sections to 39 weeks or later for this very reason.[7]
- **Breathing issues**. In addition to accidental preemies having underdeveloped lungs, full-term babies arriving by surgery can have difficulty breathing, too. C-section babies skip out on the very beneficial trip through the birth canal where contractions literally squeeze the amniotic fluid out of their lungs on their way out.
- **Risk of larger drop in baby's birth weight**. Since the excess amniotic fluid wasn't squeezed out on the baby's way out of the birth canal, the fluid, and thus, weight, is lost post-birth instead. When a baby loses more than 10 percent of his birth weight, it can send doctors into a state of worry about dehydration. This is a real concern for some babies, but for others, it's really just loss of the fluid.
- **Injury to baby**. This is rare, but still something to avoid like the plague when you're talking about your itty bitty baby getting punctured by a surgical instrument. Oww!

---

[4] More info on infant digestive tract: http://www.scienceandsensibility.org/?p=4995 and http://dralexrinehart.com/nutrition-benefits/importance-of-breastfeeding-infant-gut-development

[5] More on increased risk of allergies and asthma: http://www.ncbi.nlm.nih.gov/pubmed/16297144?report

[6] More on early births tied to C-sections: http://www.nbcnews.com/id/25193124/ns/health-pregnancy/t/rise-early-births-tied-unneeded-c-sections/#.UeGiohZUOEk

[7] More on the delay of elective C-sections to 39 weeks or later: http://healthland.time.com/2011/08/26/patience-please-39-weeks-is-the-new-thinking-about-when-to-deliver-babies

If you need a Cesarean

While it's true that major surgery is not usually the optimal way to have a baby, it *could* very well be the optimal way to have your baby, in certain circumstances. And that's really okay. There are many conditions and situations that can arise during the course of your labor that may truly necessitate a C-section. Even with all the best preparation and the most wonderful care provider and birthing team, it still happens. This can be extremely hard to swallow when you have been naturally minded all throughout your pregnancy. It's okay to feel sad about the outcome of your birth experience — even if it saved your life or your baby's life. It's really important to know that you are not a failure, and you can get support to help you grieve the loss of the experience you'd hoped for.

Also know that a C-section birth doesn't mean you can't have a family-centered and gentle experience. In most cases, a mother is under epidural anesthesia during the surgery, and so she's awake and alert. And even though mom isn't able to hold baby right away, there's no reason (unless baby is in some sort of distress) why the dad or partner can't.

Why you don't want forceps to be the driving force pulling your baby out of you

Unlike the C-section, which I suppose has its appeal what with the no immediate pain aspect and all (not taking recovery into consideration), I have yet to meet anyone who wanted a forceps-assisted delivery. This medical instrument looks like a pair of basic salad tongs. Except instead of you trying to serve up some leafy greens, your doctor is trying to serve up your infant's head. Which, by the way, is still pretty much embedded in your vagina.

An inability to push due to epidural anesthesia is one reason for needing a forceps-assisted delivery — all the more reason to avoid an epidural, but more on that later.

In all seriousness, forceps can also be linked to severe fetal injuries, and C-sections are often preferred over this operative-vaginal delivery method (which often takes place in the OR), though it could be debated which causes greater risk. It also depends on your doctor's personal experience using forceps.

A forceps delivery can also dictate the need for an episiotomy (more on that later), and can cause post-partum issues with perineal healing and urinary incontinence.[8]

Why a vacuum-assisted delivery sucks (literally)

A vacuum extraction does just that — it helps to extract a baby from mom's vagina using a small circular suction device that latches on to the baby's head while still in the birth canal. The doctor then uses a handheld pump to up the pressure applied to the head, and then pulls the baby out while the mom pushes during a contraction.[9]

As with forceps, a vacuum-assisted delivery may be used to get the baby out quickly at the end of the pushing stage for whatever reason makes it necessary. Perhaps mom has been pushing for forever and is too tired to finish the job.

Babies who come out this way often suffer from what I have officially labeled Vacuum Head, a temporary condition which makes all your otherwise adorable photos taken the first three days of life look like you gave birth to an alien. There is potential for other actual (though rare) problems to occur during this procedure as well, such as bleeding under the scalp, brain or eye injury or nerve damage.

If you're not sure which sounds worse — the doc pulling your baby out with salad tongs or yanking his head with a dust buster — they both come with similar rates of complications like vaginal trauma, tearing and incontinence, so if it comes to this, it's best to let your doctor choose whichever method he's more comfortable using.[10]

---

[8] More on forceps delivery: http://www.mayoclinic.com/health/forceps-delivery/MY02085

[9] More on vacuum delivery: http://www.mayoclinic.com/health/vacuum-extraction/MY02084

[10] Watch a vacuum demonstration:
http://www.babycenter.com/2_vacuum-and-forceps-during-birth_3656512.bc

It's worth noting that while forceps and vacuums are no picnics in the park, they can be, for some women in certain situations, their best shot at avoiding a C-section. Deciding which is preferable for you is a personal decision.

Why an episiotomy will tear you up inside (and out)

Ever wonder about that tight piece of skin that lives between your vagina and your butt? My guess is probably not. That is until someone cuts it open from end to end.

If that didn't send your spine into shivers and your kegel muscles into a panicked frenzy, then maybe you won't mind an episiotomy. But as for the rest of us, tearing in that delicate area seems almost too much to bear. Deliberately cutting it just sounds like downright cruel and unusual punishment.

I know what you're thinking. You've heard — maybe even from your obstetrician — that an artificial incision is better than a spontaneous tear because a straight cut line is easier to repair than a jagged tear one. Some argue that point (though the American Congress of Obstetricians and Gynecologists say its use should be restricted[11]). But I think I'm leaning towards keeping as much of my vag intact over making my OB's job easier.

Both natural tearing and intentional cutting of the perineum can lead to bleeding, infection, more pain, and possible sexual dysfunction. Just what you wanted to experience after your 20-hour labor is over, right? If you tear on your own, there's not much you can do about it. But you can avoid an episiotomy by simply asking your care provider to put down the scissors.

Some women who have an epidural end up having an episiotomy performed, unbeknownst to them. Because they can't feel anything from the waist down, they just have no idea what's going on. This is just another reason why it's extremely important to communicate with your care provider about your wishes before the big day (read more on that in Chapter 4).

---

[11] The American Congress of Obstetricians and Gynecologists on why episiotomies should be restricted: http://www.acog.org/About%20ACOG/News%20Room/News%20Releases/2006/ACOG%20Recommends%20Restricted%20Use%20of%20Episiotomies.aspx

There are cases where an episiotomy could become desirable; if your baby is truly in distress and needs to come out quickly, an episiotomy might be your ticket out of a potential surgery.

Why you should run, not walk, from an epidural (that is, if your legs aren't numb)

No pain during labor? The ability to sleep, carry on conversations and watch trashy TV right up until the baby is crowning? Okay, fine. I'm a natural birth advocate for sure, but I see the allure to the mighty epidural. Ask any mother who's had an epidural birth and she'll probably tell you that she loves her anesthesiologist as much as (or more than) her husband.

However, it is wise to note that those women are also peeing via catheter; are unable to get out of the bed during labor; are shivering, vomiting or both; are experiencing mild to really powerful headaches that last for hours, days, or weeks; and are, in general, not the best, most vivacious version of themselves immediately following the birth of their babies.

And those are just the superficial side effects associated with epidural anesthesia. There are real medical risks, too. Ask any one of your friends who got the magic needle in her back what those risks are, or if she was even made aware that any existed beforehand, and she is likely to have no idea that an epidural does anything but block some heavy labor pain. Unless, of course, she is one of the unlucky ones to experience one of the following epidural hazards herself:[12]

- **A slowed or stalled labor**, which can lead to the administration of synthetic oxytocin, which leads to more painful contractions, which can lead to a distressed baby, which can lead to an emergency C-section. (This scenario is known as the cascade of interventions.[13])
- **An inability to push** when it's time, which can lead to a forceps- or vacuum-assisted delivery or a C-section.
- **A drop in blood pressure**, which can lead to a distressed baby,

---

[12] More information on advantages and disadvantages of epidural:
http://www.americanpregnancy.org/labornbirth/epidural.html

[13] There is a terrific visual on the cascade of interventions based on the Listening to Mothers survey here: http://transform.childbirthconnection.org/reports/listeningtomothers/cesarean/

which can lead to an emergency C-section. (Are you noticing a pattern yet?)

- **A fever**, which can lead to a distressed baby, which can lead to an emergency C-section. Even if you manage to avoid the C-section, your baby may need a quick stop in the NICU to be sure he didn't develop an infection during your fever. He may also be given an unnecessary dose of antibiotics just in case he develops an infection.
- **Increased risk of postpartum hemorrhage**. More blood? Fun! (Not so much.)
- Really rare but serious risks include **paralysis**, **cardiac arrest** and **maternal death**. How convenient that nobody tells you about these.

Oh, and sometimes, the epidural doesn't even work! For moms whose sole birth plan is to become BFF with the anesthesiologist, it can be a pretty tough blow when she has no back-up method for dealing with the pain.

If you get an epidural

It should be noted that in some circumstances, even for a natural birthing mama, an epidural could have its place. For example, in the case of an extremely long labor, an epidural can give a tired mother a chance to rest before she has to finish the job. If for some reason an epidural becomes part of your labor's trajectory, know that you are not a failure. You can also ask that it be turned down or off after a certain period of time, so that you can resume feeling your labor and have full ability to push.

Why you'd be high to take narcotics

Ever heard a pregnant woman say she's been taking pretty serious drugs to take the edge off? Of course you haven't. That's because when you're pregnant, you can't so much as take an Advil without harming your unborn child.

Narcotics (also called opioids or analgesics) don't actually block the pain that a mom is experiencing, but rather, a mom's perception of the pain. It's kind of like when my kids are whining at dinnertime — if I have a glass of wine during the drama, it doesn't stop them from whining, but it makes me a little more patient in handling the situation.

In my dinner example, the benefits of my having a glass of wine (me smiling at my children as they fight over who gets which bowl) clearly outweigh the drawbacks (my children potentially telling their preschool teachers that Mommy's a drunk). But what about the advantages and disadvantages of narcotics during labor?

The good: You're relaxed, having a nice time, and nothing can bother you. The drugs take effect only minutes after the IV is hooked up so you get almost instant relief. Unlike the epidural, your ability to push is not disturbed, and you don't have to get a giant needle in your back.

The bad: You're drowsy, a little out of it and nauseous. It lasts for only one to several hours. It shouldn't be administered too early because it could slow your labor's progress, and it shouldn't be administered too late because it could more adversely affect your baby the closer it's given to birth. Since you're possibly dizzy and a little loopy, it's probably best that you stay in bed, which we will learn later on in Chapter 6's *Squatting: It's not just for killer quads (movement and positions during labor)*, is not best for your labor progress.

The ugly: Your breathing can be temporarily depressed. Oh, and since this stuff passes through the placenta, too, your baby could have trouble breathing as well. Even if the baby is breathing normally at birth, she still may be sleepy, and unable to breastfeed successfully due to the lasting effects of the drugs.[14]

Here's what I don't get. You spend nine months being so careful about everything you put into your body. You switch to cage-free eggs and milk from cows that haven't been treated with hormones. You spend $9 on the organic version of stretch-mark lotion just in case it seeps through your skin and into your uterus. You celebrate your birthday this year with a virgin margarita. And then, when you have less than one day to go, you throw your hands in the air and say "Eff it, give me the hard drugs." Really?

---

[14] More on narcotics: http://www.mayoclinic.com/health/labor-and-delivery/PR00105 and http://www.askdrsears.com/topics/pregnancy-childbirth/pregnancy-concerns/managing-pain-during-childbirth/narcotic-pain

Why Pitocin is the pits

Pitocin is the synthetic form of the body's naturally occurring hormone, oxytocin, which is released during childbirth. Sometimes, it's given to a woman already in labor; this is called augmentation. Other times, it's administered to a woman who is not experiencing any natural contractions; this is called induction, and in this scenario the mother may also be given other interventions to ripen her cervix as well.

Pitocin's job is to simulate contractions, and it usually gets that job done. When contractions come on their own, they typically build up slowly in frequency and in intensity. This gives the mother the wonderful gift of a paced labor where she can work through each contraction. When contractions come as a result of Pitocin, they pretty much go from zero to 60 in no time at all, and scare the bejeezus out of the laboring mother.

For someone who doesn't know much about birth yet, Pitocin sounds like a miracle drug. Get the baby out quicker? End this pain roller coaster I'm on sooner? Sign me up! But, as is the case with any labor intervention, there can be a price to pay the Pitocin Piper.

Here are the risks associated with Pitocin, as listed on the waiver that you'll likely have to sign before it's administered:

- Increased risk of infection in your baby
- Increased risk of infection in mother
- Hemorrhage (excessive bleeding)
- Increased need for Cesarean section

Sounds super, right? How's a slow and steady birth sounding now?

If you need Pitocin

If you are dealt the unfortunate Pitocin card for circumstances beyond your control (happened to me when my water broke and I was not at all in labor after 36 hours), know that you have the right to ask for as little of the medication as possible. Ask how much they normally give and then tell them you want only half. When the nurse comes in to up the dose every so often, you can ask her to skip it one time, or to increase it by only a smidge. Remember, even if an intervention becomes inevitable, you still have a say in your birth experience. Oh, and it IS possible to birth without pain meds even if you're on Pit.

Why constant electronic fetal monitoring is a constant pain in the ass

If you have an epidural or Pitocin (or other conditions that require it), you must also have constant electronic fetal monitoring, or EFM, throughout the course of your labor. Even if you don't have circumstances that ostensibly require it, EFM is standard policy in some hospitals or with some providers, which you can learn about in advance (and you can certainly request not to have it even then).

The EFM was invented in 1958, and a wonderful invention it was. With the new tool, which involves two large belts that wrap around your belly — one to monitor the heartbeat of your baby and the other to monitor your contractions — doctors could detect problems in unborn babies of high-risk mothers in enough time to do something about it. And guess what? Outcomes improved. Awesome!

What happened next is not so awesome. EFM became the standard of care in hospitals, not only for women in high-risk obstetrical circumstances, but for everyone. Now you are wondering, why does this matter? More monitoring equals more babies saved, right? Not necessarily.

Constant monitoring where every blip of the baby's heart rate is seen and recorded can sometimes result in unwarranted anxiety among the medical team members (and probably your partner as well, who will be totally enthralled by this technology like it's his new personal gadget).

Heart rates are allowed to ebb and flow and experience normal variation throughout the course of labor. A shift in heart rate does not automatically mean the baby needs to get out immediately, but the constant monitoring has led to this not-actually-distressed-baby phenomenon.

The giant EFM belts make it all but impossible to get out of the bed, so women restricted by it often stay in one horizontal position throughout their labor. Not moving around makes contractions a lot harder to manage, and so then an epidural becomes pretty inevitable (and we know why we don't want that; if you don't, then you are skimming this chapter and you need to go back and read in more detail).

EFMs are popular among hospital staff because it allows just one L&D nurse to care for four or five women at a time — she can just read the constant displays of fetal heartbeats coming in to her at the nurses' station instead of actually hanging out with a woman having a baby to, you know, support her and stuff. Imagine the cost savings for the hospital if they need only one nurse to assist with several women instead of one nurse for each and every laboring woman! The problem here is that even when the nurse manages to make her way from the nurses' station into an individual's laboring room, she often goes straight to the EFM machine, and stands there folding yards and yards of the print-out like an accordion (don't get me started on all the trees we are wasting in this mess). No "How are you doing?" or "Can I get you anything to make you more comfortable?" Nope, she just checks the machine and goes on her merry way to the next machine, er, I mean patient.

Intermittent monitoring with a Doppler (or even with an EFM for 15 minutes every hour) is usually sufficient for low-risk mothers who have not already been troubled with other interventions like an epidural or Pitocin that make the EFM required.[15]

If you need EFM

If you find yourself in a situation that requires EFM, know that you can still own this birth. Ask your care provider if you can take short breaks from EFM so that you can get out of bed and stretch, walk around, or go to the bathroom. You may even be able to wear the EFM belts while standing up and staying close to the machines to which you're tethered.

---

[15] More information on EFM: http://www.instituteofmidwifery.org/MSFinalProj.nsf/a9ee58d7a82 396768525684f0056be8d/1e5626880167e040852569fc00610cf3?OpenDocument

Why someone breaking your waters might also break your spirit

A doctor or midwife can perform this procedure using a plastic hook (which looks like a crochet hook) that is inserted into the vagina to puncture the membranes. Some women don't mind the slight discomfort of this procedure while others report pain.

The main reason your care provider might want to break your bag of waters (the medical term is artificial rupture of membranes or AROM) is to speed up your labor. The idea supporting this practice is that it will release prostaglandins, the hormones that help to ripen the cervix. It will also remove the barrier between the baby's head and the cervix, thus creating more direct pressure. Sometimes, after a woman's waters are broken for her, labor is immediately accelerated; other times, AROM will have only marginal effects. In the first scenario, contractions instantaneously become intense, which is not ideal because it doesn't give you time to naturally build up your tolerance. When contractions steadily increase in their intensity over a long time, you are better able to handle them. In the latter scenario where labor doesn't accelerate after AROM, the intervention didn't have its intended effect and was therefore done for absolutely no reason.

The most serious risk of AROM is umbilical cord prolapse, where the cord comes out ahead of baby, presenting grave danger to the baby. Breaking the waters too early can also lead to a head-first baby turning into a breech position, which will lead you straight to the operating room, though that scenario is not likely.

Those sobering risks aside, as a matter of principle, I try not to stick sharp objects up my va-jay-jay. I would also avoid the artificial rupture of membranes for more practical reasons.

It is largely believed by the medical community that once your water is broken, either on its own or artificially, your risk of infection increases. There is a range of opinion on this, so it's important to know where your care provider stands on this issue (before the big day). Some doctors will want you to come to the hospital immediately after your water breaks on its own, while others will allow you to hang out at home for a while until labor really gets started. In either case, your doctor and/or hospital has a number of hours that they will allow you to stay pregnant with ruptured membranes. For some, this number is 12 or 24; for others, like the hospital where I gave birth, the number is 48.

The point is, once your water breaks, you are on The Clock. And as someone who has been on The Clock, I can tell you, it's not a great place to be. Suddenly, there is a lot of pressure to get your contractions going, to make progress, to be in active labor, to dilate, to efface, to get the baby out, to decorate the nursery, to save for college…are you stressed out yet?

Know what happens when you're stressed out about trying to be in a good labor pattern? You get all tense and subconsciously suck in your vagina muscles in a last-ditch effort to not have this baby after all. And thus begins the cascade of interventions I mentioned earlier…Pitocin, epidural, C-section.

If your water breaks naturally, there's not much you can do about being on The Clock, short of lying to your care provider about the time it actually happened (though I don't recommend that strategy). But allowing your doctor to break your bag of waters for you? Why would you *willingly* get on The Clock?

Most women will blindly take the suggestion of AROM from their OB as an end-all mandate — something they feel they have to do for the sake of their babies' safety. But most of the time, the proposal of breaking your water is simply that — a proposal. Something that *may* speed up your labor (don't get me wrong; it might). But it will also put you on The Clock, and once you're on The Clock, you better hope your labor does in fact come on in a hurry, before you are declared a "failure to progress" and off to the operating room you go for a surgical birth.

If they need to break your water

Just like with the epidural, in certain conditions, a care provider breaking your water might not be as terrible as I just described. For example, if your labor is active and your cervix has been dilating steadily, but then suddenly your progress stops and doesn't seem to be picking up anytime soon, AROM might be a way to encourage your labor to resume. In this example, you may have just saved yourself from a C-section. If you do have your waters broken for you, it's best to wait till the baby is engaged (low down in the pelvis). And know that ruptured membranes often means you'll be getting antibiotics as well.

Are you a natural-birth groupie yet?

So there you have it — why not-so-natural birth is about as much fun as a root canal. Are you ready to sign up for your only other option?

Not only does un-natural birth suck the big one, but natural birth is actually pretty amazing. In addition to not experiencing all the horrible realities of many labor interventions, there are in fact some kick-ass side effects to natural birth.

- **Birther's high**. Of course you've heard of a runner's high. I'm a runner — with one marathon and many half marathons under my belt — so I know me some good runner's high. My birther's high was like crossing the finish line of my marathon, only birth took me about twice as long to complete and felt 100 times better. This type of high lasts for weeks, and leaves you wanting to get knocked up again as soon as possible just so you can experience it again. Natural birth is like crack for your vagina.
- **Instant recovery**. As in, you are up and walking your natural-birthing bad ass to the bathroom not long after the last push. This isn't to say that it doesn't feel like someone whacked you in the crotch with a baseball bat during that walk, but you are able to get out of bed and to the facilities to squirt water out of an old-style ketchup container directly onto your labia majora all by your lonesome, which is especially nice if you were just spread-eagle in front of an entourage of hospital personnel for the good part of the last three hours.
- **Super alert, nursing-like-a-champ baby**. You are much less likely to experience early breastfeeding hurdles if you avoided medication during labor. Your baby will come out with eyes wide open, ready to look at this awesome specimen of a mommy that just got her through the birth canal like no other, with her mouth wide open, ready to wrap little wet lips around your areola. (I feel a little bit like

I'm writing erotica right now, but I swear it's not my intention.)

- **Bragging rights**. Maybe this isn't the right reason to have a natural birth, but it is a pretty cool byproduct. I especially love it when it comes up in conversation with someone who doesn't already know that I'm a natural birth enthusiast. Because natural birth has become so rare in this country, it's so unexpected and people are genuinely impressed. When my husband goes on to say that he actually caught the baby himself ("You mean the doctor didn't deliver her?!"), the crowd goes wild.

What you just learned

- All the reasons why natural birth kicks not-natural birth's ass
- How some of the interventions we are trying to avoid may rear their ugly heads in our births and why that's okay

CHAPTER 2
Where is this birth going down?
(Choosing a birthplace)

"Have the medical team on board [and] know they'll be honest with you if things don't go as planned." — Shannon Snow, who birthed naturally in a tub as she had hoped.

Now that you're totally on board with birthing your spawn the way nature intended, this chapter is likely the most important one you'll read. Choosing a care provider and birthplace is the single biggest factor in the trajectory of your birth experience. If you choose wisely, you won't have to put much effort into other things.

I started out my first pregnancy journey much like yours, I'm sure. I was seeing my OB/GYN once a month for an appointment where I would wait in the lobby for about 45 minutes first, and then she would see me in the exam room for approximately two minutes where she would proclaim everything was moving along fine and I could see her again in a month.

Up until about 20 weeks along, I had very surface-type thoughts about natural childbirth. I basically figured I would try my best not to succumb to the epidural for as long as I could, but I reserved my right to change my mind at any given time. (Does this sound familiar? Keep reading.)

At about 15 weeks into my pregnancy, my husband and I attended a Christmas party. A woman there who was also pregnant (her second) and who, unbeknownst to me at the time, was a natural birth enthusiast asked me if I intended to birth naturally. I told her I wanted to, but that I would make a game-time decision. She asked where I was delivering, and I named the hospital with which my OB was affiliated. Then she said, with very matter-of-fact certainty, "Oh, you're going to get an epidural *there*."

I had no idea what she meant by that. Somehow the place of my birth dictated whether or not I'd need pain relief? Had I chosen a hospital that would make my labor hurt more? I shrugged off her comment as mere rudeness. How was she so sure I'd surrender to the drugs? *Well, I'd show her,* I thought. At least, I would *try* to show her, and then I'd see how much it hurt, and then I'd make a decision. Yeah, that was my plan.

I also had no idea that her remark, and what would come next, would change my life. Soon after the holiday party, she passed along a DVD, Ricki Lake's documentary, *The Business of Being Born*, to her husband to give to my husband.

After he watched it, my otherwise smart husband said, "I think you should give birth naturally."

Oh really? "I think YOU should give birth naturally," I replied. Then he talked me into watching the documentary by bribing me with a foot rub. Now, years later, it's hard for me to separate out what I initially took away from that first viewing, and what I would later learn reading dozens of books and articles, and eventually the sequels to Ricki's first documentary. But I remember that I watched it twice in one weekend, and that I cried both times I saw the scene where Ricki, naked in her bathtub, reaches down to catch her own baby.

It was like nothing I'd ever seen before (and I recommend you go watch this must-see feature as soon as you are finished reading this book). Suddenly I couldn't learn enough about natural birth. I was hooked.

After watching this film I went into immediate research mode. Here are a few things I picked up:

- Birth is a business; hospitals make money off of you giving birth. They make more money if you have a C-section instead of a vaginal delivery.
- Hospitals have policies in place that are, in general, in the best interest of the hospital, not of the patient. These policies largely serve the purpose of preventing a scenario in which the hospital or doctor is sued.
- With these policies often comes a cascade of medical interventions.
- In hospitals, laboring women are encouraged to have an epidural

because they are more "manageable" or require less one-on-one care when they aren't bothered with the pains of labor. Epidurals are often the first step in the cascade of interventions.

- The ultimate intervention is a C-section. The C-section rate in this country was about 32 percent in 2009, 2010 and 2011.[16] The recommended rate by the World Health Organization is 5-10 percent with an upward limit of 15 percent.[17]

- Midwives are a great alternative to obstetricians. Obstetricians are trained to see pathology (i.e. medical emergency, crisis, danger). Midwives are trained in normal, physiological birth. They are oftentimes more patient in letting labor take its natural course, and are less focused on arbitrary rules about how long labor should last or in what position a mother should have to push.

What are my birthplace choices?

If you are reading this book, then you're probably already pregnant, and you've likely already chosen a hospital as the place in which your child will enter this world. Even so, as with everything else in birth, it's always better to know all your options, and be armed with that knowledge. It is also of note that it is only too late to switch hospitals or providers *after the baby is born*. If you are 41 weeks pregnant, but indeed still pregnant, you can still make a switch. That is not an exaggeration or a joke. As long as you are still pregnant, you can still switch to a care provider or birthplace that more closely meets your needs.

After *The Business of Being Born* changed my perspective, I reexamined my initial choice of hospital and care provider and made a switch.

Home birth

Let's begin with the home. As in *your* home. As in you can squat down right where you are right now, on your bed or in the middle of your living room floor and pop a baby out.

---

[16] More stats from the Centers for Disease Control and Prevention here: http://www.cdc.gov/nchs/data/databriefs/db124.htm

[17] More Birth by the Numbers stats here: http://www.birthbythenumbers.org

When I first became pregnant and hadn't yet delved into this arena of natural birth, I honestly had never even heard of home birth. I definitely didn't know anyone who'd had one or was planning one. It seemed really archaic and unsafe. I thought home birth was what people did before there were hospitals.

I thought, isn't it better to have all the technology that is available in this day and age within arm's reach? And why would anyone want to get all the blood and whatever else comes out on the 800-thread-count sheets that you got for your bridal shower just a few years back?

But what is home birth exactly? In the case of a planned home birth, a pregnant woman hires a midwife. Depending on your state's laws, you may be required to hire only a certified nurse-midwife (CNM), but other states will allow certified professional midwives (CPMs) to attend home births.[18] Currently, CPMs are legal in only 28 states. In the other 22 states, as well as the District of Columbia, a CPM is at risk for criminal prosecution if she practices midwifery. This conundrum can make it very difficult to have a home birth in those states because you'll be hard-pressed to find a private midwife to attend the birth.

But if you live in a state with CPM licensing, or if you can secure a CNM to attend your birth, the midwife will come to your home to take care of all of your prenatal appointments (sounds pretty convenient!). You may still choose to have all the prenatal tests available at facilities near you that offer sonograms and blood tests, etc.

One potential downside to a home birth is the lack of insurance coverage. Where your insurance is likely to cover all or nearly all of your hospital birth costs, it most likely will not cover the expense of a private midwife performing your prenatal care and attending your home delivery. Out-of-pocket costs can range from $2,000 to $6,000 or more, depending on the provider and where you live. Some midwives will offer a sliding scale based on your ability to pay. It also may be possible to get your insurance to cover part of the bill if they see your midwife simply as an out-of-network provider. And some insurance plans will cover home birth, but that is the

---

[18] More on a campaign to support the expansion of out-of-hospital maternity care and certified professional midwives in all 50 states: http://pushformidwives.org

exception and not the rule. It's worth the time and effort to write your insurance company a letter to explain to them why they should cover the cost of your home birth, i.e. how they will ultimately save money by you giving birth at home, because it's less costly than a hospital delivery.

When it comes time and labor begins, you will alert your midwife, and she will assess, usually by talking to you on the phone, what stage of labor you are in and if she needs to rush over. More likely, she can wait a while. At some point, you both determine that she is needed, and she comes to your house. She monitors you and the baby, and stays with you or around you throughout the rest of your labor. The constant presence of your medical attendant is an important point that differentiates a home birth from a hospital birth.

A midwife typically follows a hands-off approach to a laboring woman, allowing your body and your baby to control the course of your labor. That could mean your labor takes a couple of hours, or a couple of days. But, barring the incidence of a medical necessity, you are free to labor however you see fit: in the tub, in the shower, drinking water, eating a cheeseburger, in the nude, bundled up in a blanket, walking around, climbing stairs, in the bed, standing up, squatting. *You* are in charge.

And contrary to what my naïve self may have thought, it turns out, studies show that home birth is *just as safe* as hospital birth for low-risk pregnancies (and some would argue it's actually safer[19]). Now, there certainly is much controversy on this matter, and you could find studies to back up whatever your personal opinion happens to be. If you talk to an EMT or an OB about home birth, they are likely to tell you about all the home-birth-gone-wrong scenarios they have personally witnessed, and the horror that ensued. The problem with their points of view is that they only see the incidents of home birth that have required a transfer to the hospital. When a home birth goes smoothly, as it often does, the only people who see it are mom, dad and the midwife (and maybe big brother or sister and the dog).

Anyone interested should do her own research on home birth, and draw her own conclusions about whether it's right for her and her family.

---

[19] More on the safety of home birth in low-risk pregnancies: http://www.bmj.com/content/346/bmj.f3263

With regard to natural birth though, staying home is definitely the best bet for success. No one will pressure you to get an epidural (it's not available even if you decide you want it!) and no one will suggest surgery unless it is truly necessary (again, not available, and would require a transfer to the hospital). And no one can argue you on that point.

For me, pregnant with my first baby and just beginning to reexamine my birthplace options, I didn't spend much time considering home birth. Don't get me wrong; the more I read about it, the more I was intrigued, and the less "out there" it seemed. But as a first-timer just learning about everything, I didn't think my townhouse that shared walls with the neighbors was the best fit for my moaning-and-groaning natural-birth party. My husband was also, like many first-time dads might be, not crazy about the idea, and felt more confident in a setting that didn't involve our leather sofa.

If you overcome the basic heebie jeebies about giving birth at home, you also need to check with your care provider to see if you'd be a candidate for home birth. Certain factors or complications may make a home birth too risky, and these circumstances might be different depending on what care provider you ask. So if you ask your hospital-based obstetrician if you can deliver your breech twins at home, you may get a different answer from the one you'll get if you ask the home-birth midwife who'd actually be attending it.

Birth center

The next option, which, prior to being pregnant, I also had never heard of, is a birth center. Often affiliated or even physically connected to a hospital, this alternative gives moms the best of both worlds — a home-like setting with medical interventions out of the delivery room, but only a stone's throw away when needed.

And unlike a home birth, birth center deliveries are usually covered by insurance the same way they would be in a hospital, due to the center's relationship with a hospital and with physicians.

When I first learned of birth centers, this immediately became an attractive option for me. A place where I could give birth naturally, without having to defend my decisions or fight to avoid interventions, while still being close enough to the hospital for emergencies? Sign me up!

The column for pros is long on the birth center list. They handle your prenatal care at the birth center, so you are still able to get to know your provider throughout your pregnancy. Most, if not all, birthing centers provide birthing tubs so you have the option for a water birth. As with home birth, there aren't any restrictions surrounding your labor movement, birth position, what you can eat, who can be there, and if you can take pictures or video. The technology for monitoring you and the baby, and even for providing certain types of pain relief are available to you right at the birth center.

The only con for birth centers is that there just aren't enough of them. In my area, for instance (and I live near more than one metropolitan city), the closest birth center is about 45 minutes away. I could give birth at any of about 10 hospitals within 25 minutes, but if I want a room with a rug, curtains and a tub, I'd have to travel nearly an hour (and for all my prenatal appointments, too). Given the distance, I steered away from the birth center route, and set about finding the right hospital to birth my baby.

Hospital

The idea of home birth, at the beginning of my journey, seemed a little too ambitious for me, and definitely for my husband, who wouldn't even entertain the idea. Now that I'm a natural birth junkie (maybe you'll get there one day, too), hearing and reading about home birth is very commonplace and doesn't make me bat an eyelash. And yet I still have some reservations about it for me personally.

The truth is that, by and large, most births go relatively smoothly, leaving just a small percentage where some type of emergency happens, and a physician and operating room become urgent and necessary.

Sometimes, in those cases — the ones where something goes awry — there is time to call an ambulance or even drive to the hospital going the legal speed limit. But there are a few circumstances where that is not the case, when the hospital is just a few too many minutes away for a successful-outcome transfer.

One article suggests that the following four conditions are the only ones better handled at the hospital than at home[20]:

1. Cord prolapse (where the cord is in front of the baby on its way out; happens less than 1 percent of the time[21])

2. Ruptured uterus (a tear in the uterine wall; happens 1-2 percent of the time in women attempting a VBAC (vaginal birth after cesarean)[22]; I couldn't even find statistics on women never having had a C-section because they are so low)

3. Amniotic fluid embolism (where amniotic fluid gets into the mother's bloodstream during or right after birth; happens at a rate so far below 1 percent that I could barely count the number of zeros that go after the decimal point[23])

4. Placental abruption (when the placenta peels away from the uterus before the baby is born; happens 1 percent of the time worldwide[24])

And while the statistics on those or other rare but serious conditions may be miniscule, for me, it was still too hard to process the idea that, should I end up as one of the unlucky few, I wouldn't have made the right decision for my baby.

A longtime friend of mine had an uncomplicated hospital birth with her first baby, and was planning for the same with her second a few years later. Unfortunately, things don't always go as planned, and her placenta unexpectedly detached while she was in labor. Luckily, she was in the hospital when she needed an emergency C-section. They got her little boy out in three minutes. Had she been farther away from the operating room, there would not have been time, and her son may not have survived.

---

[20] More on all of these emergencies:
http://www.greenmedinfo.com/blog/myth-safer-hospital-birth-low-risk-pregnancies

[21] More on cord prolapse:
http://my.clevelandclinic.org/healthy_living/pregnancy/hic_umbilical_cord_prolapse.aspx

[22] More on uterine rupture:
http://www.vbac.com/what-is-a-uterine-rupture-and-how-often-does-it-occur/

[23] More on amniotic fluid embolism:
http://www.mayoclinic.com/health/amniotic-fluid-embolism/DS01207

[24] More on placental abruption: http://www.mayoclinic.com/health/placental-abruption/DS00623

I don't tell you this story to scare you. And I'm not saying that I'm against home birth or birth center birth. I'm actually a huge proponent for both. Prior to this scary incident that hit so close to home for me, I'd only heard accounts of cases where, yeah, a birth ended in a C-section, but it wasn't like a running-through-the-hospital-while-your-husband-happened-to-be-in-the-cafeteria-but-it-doesn't-matter-just-get-the-baby-out-NOW kind of circumstance. This was the first birth story I'd been told where it was truly a life-or-death matter where every minute counted and being in the hospital saved her baby's life, and possibly her own, too.

Okay, you got through reading that scary story. You can stop holding your breath now. Here's another, less frightening one for you. My first baby came as a surprise at 34 weeks (he was totally fine, by the way, just tiny. Read entire story in the "My Own Birth Stories" section at the end of the book). If I had been hoping for a home birth, or even a birth center birth for that matter, I would not have been able to carry out that arrangement as planned, since a baby of that gestation needs immediate care by NICU staff. Unlike my friend, I had plenty of warning to get to a hospital, so even if I had been planning to stay home, when my water broke at 33 weeks and 6 days, I would have known to go to a hospital instead.

But I was glad that the hospital was my Plan A. I got to be cared for by the team of midwives whom I'd gotten to know throughout my pregnancy, not some random OB who I just met that day who didn't know or care about my plan for a natural birth. And I wasn't dealing with the disappointment of having to birth in a hospital on top of everything else I was dealing with that day.

So if the hospital is your choice birthplace from the get-go, I am totally with you. Home births and birth center births are wonderful, and I am so grateful that they are options for the women who want them. I am even a little envious of the women who are confident and strong enough to have them. I think giving birth in my own home would be the ultimate experience for bringing a child into my family. And if I could be guaranteed a seamless and uneventful event, I might even be brave enough to talk my hubby into it.

But for me, and maybe for you, too, with the unknown factors that birth can present a tiny fraction of the time, the hospital offered me the opportunity to unleash my baby from my womb without having to worry that if something went wrong — if I were in that small percentage — that I didn't make the right choice.

And we are not alone in that thinking. In the United States, the hospital is the obvious option for most women. While home births increased 29 percent from 2004 to 2009, accounting for 29,650 of 4.2 million, or less than three-quarters of one percent of U.S. births (according to a study from the Centers for Disease Control and Prevention released in May 2011), still more than 4.1 million mothers chose the hospital.[25]

What you just learned

- You have choices in where you give birth
- Each of those choices has advantages and disadvantages
- You need to sit down with your partner and choose what's right for you and for this birth

---

[25] More on the rise of home birth: http://www.cdc.gov/nchs/data/databriefs/db84.pdf

CHAPTER 3

Wisely choosing a hospital and a care provider

"Line up everything you can in a situation [such as birth] where you don't have control. Know it can go a million different ways."—Rebecca Teaff, who says she had a "picture-perfect hospital natural experience" which would not have happened if she hadn't prepared. Rebecca switched care providers and hospitals after becoming pregnant. Even though she loved her doctor who had even helped her become pregnant with fertility treatments, she knew the C-section rate at his affiliated hospital was higher than she was comfortable with.

"Be comfortable with your practice and your OB or midwife."—Rachel Rossbach, who birthed vaginally with an epidural that she let wear off before it was time to push. When her midwife recommended she get an epidural that would allow her to sleep after a couple of long days of labor and no rest, this mom-to-be felt confident that the midwife had her best interests in mind. She had switched from an OB practice more than halfway through her pregnancy; one she ran from when her doctor asked her why she would ever consider giving birth without an epidural. Good thinking!

A lot of die-hards in the natural birth community can seem anti-hospital. They may have had a personal bad experience in the hospital, which then led them on their path to the natural birth world, and now they see the home as the only safe option where they won't be pressured to yield to the medical interventions that made them dissatisfied with their first experience. I don't disbelieve that those women had a less-than-ideal encounter at the hospital. That happens all the time. But I do believe that positive, natural births can take place at the hospital for those who wish to welcome their babies there.

The key is finding the right hospital

Allow me to repeat for emphasis, *the key is finding the right hospital*.

If you choose to birth in your home or at a birth center, your odds for achieving a natural birth are in your favor. Given the lack of anesthesiologists and serious drugs on site, you basically *have* to have a natural birth in either of these locations. You'd have to transport to the hospital not to.

But for women who want to give birth in the hospital, the odds of an unmedicated, intervention-free birth are not in their favor. This doesn't mean you can't do it. When I first found out I was pregnant, I already had an OB/GYN who was affiliated with a hospital where I knew many friends and relatives had given birth (it should have been a red flag that most of them had C-sections there but it wasn't on my radar at the time). It did not even cross my mind to reconsider my place of birth, at first. But once I realized that birth was something to be researched and carefully planned (well, the parts you can plan, anyway), my choice of care provider and affiliated hospital were the first things I reexamined.

If you haven't yet made a conscious decision about your care provider and place of birth, here are some questions to ask at your next appointment (or in an interview appointment, if you are shopping around for a new provider). I've provided commentary about what would be ideal or acceptable answers to me, but these may differ for you personally.

1. **What is the C-section rate at this hospital? What is this practice's rate?** (Note: the national average in recent years was 32-33 percent, and you can check this website to see if the hospi-

tal's rate is listed: www.cesareanrates.com/hospital-level-cesare-an-rates.) **What is the C-section rate for first-time moms?** (Note: this might be more relevant since it eliminates the many repeat C-section moms, though it may be harder to nail down this statistic.) I would not feel comfortable at a hospital whose rate is higher than the national average. If you can find a midwife practice, you may find their practice's rate to be significantly lower than their affiliated hospital's rate. Note that midwives don't perform the C-sections themselves, but cases where their patients' births ended up in surgery would be counted as a C-section outcome.

2. **What were the reasons for your last five C-section deliveries?**

    a. **"Failure to progress"** is a common reason for a C-section, but not an acceptable one in my book. In essence, this means that the care provider experienced "failure to wait long enough" since each woman's labor is completely unique, and there is no set time for how long it should take. Granted, other factors may be at play here causing a woman's labor to stall, even if her care provider is patient. But some of those are preventable, such as avoiding an epidural that may slow down contractions, or eliminating unnecessary people in the room who may inadvertently cause the laboring woman to subconsciously suspend contractions (more on this later in this chapter under "Tell everyone to leave" and in Chapter 6). Failure to progress can also be a red flag for a posterior position (the back of the baby's head is towards mom's back), and moving positions can change this (you can also ask your care provider about seeing a chiropractor during pregnancy).

    b. **Previous C-section** is also a popular cause for a repeat surgery. It would be important for me to know if the mothers were choosing the C-section themselves after being educated about their choices, or if the care provider was presenting the repeat surgery as the only option. This is not a book about VBAC (vaginal birth after cesarean), but it wouldn't hurt to go with an OB/midwife who supports a woman's right to choose a VBAC.

    c. **"The baby was too big."** This is a tough one. I'm no doctor, but I know from my own personal experience that vaginas are like stretchy, elastic rubber bands (and they do eventually go back to normal, pre-stretched size, I promise). They were made to stretch. They literally were built for the purpose of birthing babies. So why would they be constructed to stretch open just a liiiiitttttle bit too small for a baby to pass through? Now, there are rare cases where a woman's pelvis really is too narrow to safely birth her baby. But these cases are the extreme exceptions, reserved for women with nutritional deficiencies, past back surgery or spinal fusion, or past break of tailbox/coocyx. If you are petite, this does not mean that your pelvis is too small to birth your baby. If your husband is substantially taller/larger than you, this does not mean that your pelvis is too small to birth his baby. A skilled care provider will be able to show you optimal positions for encouraging a large baby down and out of the birth canal. Hint: gravity is your friend.

d. **Twins.** As long as Baby A is head-down, a woman pregnant with twins should be able to birth them both vaginally. I believe that automatic C-sections for the sole reason of twins is not how our birth system should operate (pun intended) in this country. But I do understand that a multiples birth comes with its own risks, and with the way hospitals are run as a business, it doesn't surprise me. And I don't fault women who don't know to question their doctors' recommendation (or should I say instruction) to have the automatic surgery.

e. **Breech or malposition**, where the baby's head is not down and ready to come out first (there are different variations: bottom first, feet first, knees first, sideways/transverse; not all of these are possible to even attempt vaginally). It's hard to find a care provider at a hospital, and sometimes even a midwife at home, willing to deliver your breech baby. There are two reasons for this. **Number one**: There is just too much legal and financial risk for that provider to take when it's much easier for them to perform a C-section right off the bat. C-sections come with risks, too, but it's easier for the doctor to prove he "did everything he could" when he was already performing the surgery. **Number two**: Doctors just aren't taught how to vaginally deliver breech babies anymore. They are taught to perform C-sections for them instead. I personally wouldn't want an untrained doctor delivering my breech baby, so if I couldn't find a qualified professional in a hospital setting willing to try, I would opt for surgery myself (at least for a first baby; some care providers will allow a vaginal breech delivery after at least one prior head-first vaginal delivery). Note that there are ways to try to turn a breech baby before it's time for delivery, but it gets harder the further along you are in your pregnancy, so ask your provider to observe your baby's probable position at your prenatal appointments. If your baby is not in the proper position, visit a chiropractor and check out www.spinningbabies.com.

f. **Fetal distress.** This is a real reason. This C-section may have saved this baby's life. Whether the fetal distress came on naturally or was brought on by elective medical interventions is a different question. Either way, you don't want your baby to be in distress. Of course, distress typically comes on gradually and not suddenly, and there are techniques you can use (like changing position) before immediately turning to surgery.

g. **Other complications or emergencies that arise.** The mother is diabetic or has high blood pressure. An occurrence of placenta previa or other placental obstacles. These are all real reasons for a C-section, no question.

3. **What were the reasons for your last five inductions and/or augmentations?** (Induction is when a woman is not in labor and is administered drugs, such as Pitocin, to artificially induce labor; augmentation is when a woman is already in labor, and is administered drugs to speed up a labor that has slowed down or isn't progressing as quickly as a care provider would like to see.)

a. **An overdue baby.** Your baby is not a library book. You're not going to have to pay a fine if she comes out past 40 weeks. While there may be some real dangers to a very postdates baby (as in 42 weeks or more), the perceived risks of carrying a baby beyond the estimated due date just aren't accurate. A due date is calculated by your menstrual cycle, not even by the date of conception. Many women know exactly when they conceived, and yet are given a due date based on an entirely different set of rules. This is fine for estimation purposes, but when it comes down to the wire, and your induction-happy doctor thinks you're 41 weeks, and maybe you're really only 40 weeks, it can become a problem. A normal pregnancy lasts 38-42 weeks but that doesn't mean that the majority last 40 weeks. In fact, for first-time moms, the median length of pregnancy is 41 weeks and 1 day; and for a seasoned mom, 40 weeks and 3 days.[26] Ask the care provider in question how "overdue" was their patient who was induced, and what the hospital or practice policies are on this topic. Some allow women to go until 41 weeks; others will hold off on induction until 42.

b. **"The baby was getting too big."** Here we go again. What's with all these ginormous babies taking residence in these tiny uteri, unable to do the exact job they were designed to do (that job being to carry them and then birth them)? Fetal macrosomia is an actual condition when your baby is in fact too large for its gestational age, but it can't be diagnosed until after birth.[27] Often a woman will be induced for a baby that seemed too large according to its sonogram weight estimation (which are notoriously inaccurate[28]), but then ends up emerging into this world a completely healthy and normal weight. Also keep in mind that the baby's overall weight isn't always the most important factor in determining if a baby will be too large to come out; the size of the head is much more critical than how much squishy baby fat surrounds the arms and legs. Squishy arms, legs and belly just slide right out of there (and don't underestimate the power of the giant tub of KY Jelly they will use to ease the head out either; that stuff is fierce).

c. **Ruptured membranes**. A woman whose waters have broken does not automatically require an augmented labor, and yet some women who come to the hospital leaking fluid from their lady parts are instantly hooked up to Pitocin. Why? Research done in the 1960s determined that it was unsafe for a laboring woman to have ruptured membranes beyond 24 hours. Studies showed that an infection was more likely to develop after that point. However, this research didn't take enough information into account; among the design flaws, the study included women who were both term

---

[26] A study on "The length of uncomplicated human gestation": http://www.ncbi.nlm.nih.gov/pubmed/2342739

[27] More on macrosomia: http://www.mayoclinic.com/health/fetal-macrosomia/DS01202/DSECTION=tests-and-diagnosis

[28] A study: "A systematic review of the ultrasound estimation of fetal weight": http://onlinelibrary.wiley.com/doi/10.1002/uog.1751/abstract

and pre-term, even though their risk for infection varies greatly.[29] So some doctors and hospitals have become obsessed with that number, and use it as a fast and hard rule, instead of as a general guide. Your head won't explode if your water is broken for 24 hours and 2 minutes (I happen to know from personal experience that it won't happen after 47 hours either). As long as you and your baby are monitored either by yourself at home (just make sure baby continues to move and you don't develop a fever) or by your care providers at the hospital, you have plenty of time to have your baby without the use of artificial assistance. If your labor is progressing steadily, you will eventually have your baby. No need to speed up the process if there is no medical indication beyond the fact that your water broke. But if the fluid coming out of you is not clear, or if you are pre-term (before 37 weeks), tell your care provider right away. And if there is any indication that the umbilical cord is on its way out ahead of the baby (if you can see it coming out or you can feel it with your hands), call 911.

d. **Elective inductions**, based on a doctor's work schedule or out-of-town grandparents' visits aren't acceptable reasons to induce in my book. Maybe the provider wasn't the one who suggested the induction; maybe the mother herself proposed a particular birth date to coincide with her favorite aunt's birthday or the day when she'd have a convenient babysitter for her toddler. But it's the care provider's responsibility to tell her patients what is medically necessary and best for them and for their babies. And excluding medical reasons, it's best for the baby to choose his or her own birthday. Period. I'd think twice before moving forward with a care provider who haphazardly allows her patients to dictate medical decisions. What if the patient is 39 or 40 weeks already, you ask? Then it can't possibly matter, can it? As I mentioned before, your due date is just an estimate. So 39 weeks may very well be 37 weeks. You just can't know for sure. And then you've just given birth to a barely term baby, for no good reason. And induction doesn't come without its complications, so you really don't want to have one for any non-medical reasons (go back to Chapter 1 and read *Why Pitocin is*

---

[29] More on ruptured membranes and the risk of infection:
http://www.medscape.com/viewarticle/494127

the pits).

e. **Pre-existing conditions in mother or baby** that indicate an induction is necessary. Diabetes, pre-eclampsia, high blood pressure, a baby who has stopped growing. Totally legitimate. Induce away.

4. **How quickly should I come to the hospital after my water breaks?** Unless 1) you are less than 37 weeks along, 2) the fluid you are leaking isn't clear in color, 3) there is presence of the umbilical cord or 4) you are Group B Strep positive (a test you will have done at around 36 weeks), there is absolutely no rush to go to the hospital just because your water has broken. If any of those four scenarios are true, you'll want to get to the hospital sooner rather than later, but you still don't need to leave the house in some kind of frantic hurry with your pants around your ankles and your hair brushed only on one side (with the exception of the prolapsed cord one). Precipitous labor, also referred to as super-duper fast labor that goes from start to finish in three hours or less, isn't so common in first-time mothers, so you likely have tons of time. Stay home and labor there for a while. Eat. Sleep if you can. Do a load of laundry if you feel up to it. You can even take a shower. The only thing you can't do once your water breaks is have intercourse or put anything into your vagina. Feel free to have your husband play with your nipples though, if your labor is having a hard time beginning on its own. Run, *do not walk*, from a provider who tells you to rush to the hospital after your waters break "to get things going." That is code for augmentation.

5. **Once I'm admitted to the hospital, what policies apply?**

a. Am I allowed **freedom of movement**? What if my waters have broken? Some hospitals really restrict you once you're admitted, especially if your membranes have ruptured. You want to find a hospital that will allow you to get out of bed to use the bathroom, and to walk and move around as you see fit. Even if you have an IV for antibiotics or other drugs, you should still be permitted the freedom to walk as far as your wires and tubes will let you.

b. Am I allowed **food and drink**? Many hospitals allow absolutely nothing once you are admitted. This school of thought is based on very old-school practices. "This oral intake restriction can be traced back to the 1940s, when C-sections were performed under general anesthesia. Complications could arise if stomach contents were drawn into the lungs while under anesthesia, resulting in severe lung damage or even death. Over the years, obstetric anesthesia has become much more sophisticated. Plus, most women today receive local anesthesia for their C-sections."[30] I was caught eating a peanut butter and jelly sandwich as I was getting comfortable in my L&D room, and my nurse made a note in my file, with an attitude, I might mention, that I was consuming three bites of contraband. Some hospitals will allow you to have clear fluids, which might include water, Italian ice, chicken soup broth, and more. Giving birth is like running a marathon in a lot of ways (I've done both so I say this with personal knowledge); you need to fuel up beforehand, and you'll need some snacks in the middle to give you bursts of energy to get through it. And while this may not be my number one priority in finding the perfect hospital, a facility that is flexible in this arena is likely to be flexible and accommodating in others as well.

c. Will I have to have an **IV?** While a saline lock is policy in pretty much all hospitals (allowing easier access to your vein if the need to administer intravenous drugs later on should arise), IVs used to at least pump fluids through your veins are only required in some. Should you require fluids for a medical reason, this is nice and handy, but if it's just a precautionary measure given to everyone, there can be side effects, such as excessive weight loss for your newborn in his first three days.[31]

6. **Thinking of your last 10 births, how many episiotomies have you done and what were the reasons?** When I interviewed a midwife from the practice that I ended up switching to, she told me she couldn't remember the last episiotomy she did, and that they were not routinely performed by any midwife in the practice. This is the answer you want to hear. An even better answer would include how the care provider encourages use of alternative birthing positions to widen the pelvis and allow gravity to assist with getting the baby out.

---

[30] A study says women can eat and drink during labor:
http://summaries.cochrane.org/CD003930/eating-and-drinking-in-labour

[31] Study: "Excess weight loss in first-born breastfed newborns relates to maternal intrapartum fluid balance." http://www.ncbi.nlm.nih.gov/pubmed/21173007

7. **How many providers are in the practice?** Some OB/GYN
    offices run like a factory. One practice I used to go to took about
    10 minutes to go through each doc's name on the voicemail when
    I'd call for a simple appointment. If I had been there when I was
    pregnant, I don't know that I would have even had enough prena-
    tal appointments to meet each one once, let alone twice. Another
    practice I went to for a while was a solo practitioner. Perhaps this is
    why she was always running behind schedule — she was probably
    attending births in between other patients' office appointments.
    Given her office responsibilities and the fact that she had her own
    family and couldn't possibly be on call all the time, I determined it
    was unlikely that she'd personally be able to attend my birth, and
    I'd end up with a back-up practice OB, also known as *someone I've
    never met before.* Ultimately, I decided that neither of these scenarios
    was right for me, and the midwife practice I settled on had about six
    midwives and two obstetricians. The number was small enough that
    I was able to rotate through each of the midwives over the course
    of my pregnancy so that I'd be comfortable with whichever one was
    working at the time of my birth. The number was large enough that
    one midwife from the practice was ALWAYS working a shift at the
    hospital, so there was no chance I'd get a stranger on the big day.

8. **Is everyone in the practice aligned philosophically?** Once
    you figure out what size practice works for you, this is perhaps
    the more important question. It's unlikely that everyone will have
    completely identical opinions on everything, but it's worth the time
    to get a sense of where everyone stands on the big issues, since you
    never know which provider will be The One.

Making the hospital as home-birthy as possible

Even if you've determined that the hospital is the best place for your baby's
birth, you may still long for some aspects of a home birth. There are a few
easy ways to make your hospital experience a little less hospital-like and a
little more like home.

Wear your own clothes.

At first consideration of this idea, you might think that you don't want to get your own clothes all birthy and covered in whatever comes out in the process. For starters, I'm not suggesting you wear your favorite t-shirt or anything you may want to ever wear again. Go to a discount store, and pick yourself up a nightgown in a couple sizes larger than you normally wear. You may not even have to go to the maternity section (those may cost a little more). You can get a plain, cotton, short-sleeved nightgown for about $15. Here's why I think it's a good investment.

What could possibly feel more hospital-esque than wearing an awful hospital gown? You already feel as big as a house, but wearing a hospital gown, and maybe even two if you are up and walking around (remember, it opens in the back, so you'll need to put one on as expected and one on like a coat), I assure you, will make you feel like a McMansion. So just for basic feelings of being the best version of your pregnant self, wear your own clothes.

On a more important note, some women's labors, progressing steadily at home, upon their arrival and admittance to the hospital, will pretty much come to a screeching halt. Now, this can be attributed to a number of factors, but one of them is the general apprehension that comes from being somewhere unfamiliar. An easy way to combat this phenomenon is to make the new environment as familiar as possible. Wearing your own clothes is a good first step. If you close your eyes and feel the smooth cotton of your own budget nightgown on your skin, you can almost convince yourself that you're still in the comfort of your bedroom. (This phenomenon is less likely to occur the further you are advanced in labor.)

And on a more shallow note, hospital gowns look awful in photos. You don't want to appear sickly in your first photos with your new baby. Choose a nightgown in a color that brings out your eyes.

Bring your own tunes.

Listening to the steady, beeping rhythm of whatever contraptions they have you hooked up to — sometimes required for various reasons, even if you birth naturally — does not make for a Zen-like birth. Bring your iPod and headphones and make sure you have your birthing playlist ready to go. If you're using your phone as an iPod, turn it to airplane mode so you're not interrupted by phone calls, texts and emails.

What's on a birthing playlist? Glad you asked. Depending on what birthing class you take, you may already have a CD with birthing affirmations of some sort. If not, you can search for these in iTunes and see what suits you. When I first started listening to the affirmations (especially without my headphones so my husband was listening, too), I felt a little cheesy and a lot ridiculous. "Your body was meant to birth" and "Breathe love into your baby" the lady with the soothing voice assured me. Is she kidding me? But after I got into this way of thinking, I actually bought into all of the things the affirmation lady was saying to me, and it didn't seem so crazy after all. My body really was meant to birth! And breathing love into my baby was going to help it find its way through the birth canal!

Okay, so if you're still just not that into affirmations, your birthing soundtrack might include other soft, yoga-type music that helps to relax you or put you to sleep. You may also throw in a few songs that have personal meaning for you — the one you and your husband danced to at your wedding perhaps — or anything that will put you in the right frame of mind. Your goal is to feel relaxed, calm, confident, and, well, like your body was meant to birth. You may wish to create multiple playlists to use in different points in labor. Quiet and soothing may work early on; fast and upbeat may be just what you need for pushing.

It smells like birth in here.

Well, maybe the smell of birth isn't so bad, but the general scent of a hospital might be. Do the scents you're experiencing encourage you to relax your muscles and go into a deeper place within yourself? Or does the smell of latex rubber gloves and chemical cleaning solution disturb that ambience just a tad?

The next time you go to a yoga class (well, maybe not a bikram yoga class), and you are able to completely and totally unwind and find your inner calm, notice how your nose feels. Perhaps the instructor has lit cucumber-melon candles, or there is a lavender-scented air freshener plugged into the wall.

Whatever it is, find out, and then figure out how you can take that to the hospital with you.

The goal is to replicate the exact environment in which you have been practicing your relaxation. So if you normally close your eyes and breathe deeply while you're folding laundry, and this is how you've been preparing for birth, bring a stack of dryer sheets with you.

The power of smell is, well, powerful. It can inhibit you and it can empower you. Take note of what aromas work for you, and then stuff them in your bag.

Bring your own birth stuff.

The hospital has some equipment for you to use to aid you in getting this human out of your uterus. I use the term "equipment" loosely to mean a bed. Maybe a bar that attaches to the bed. If you're lucky, they might have a birthing tub. But it's unlikely they have other birth gear that a natural mama like you would find useful.

A birth ball. This is an easy one. It costs $5 and you may already have one, only you call it an exercise ball. It's a pain to carry into the hospital, but you'll be glad you have it to bounce or circle around on while you're in labor. And it's another place to sit besides the hospital bed, which seriously feels so hospital-y. Your partner and doula will thank you for the additional variety in seating, too.

A birthing stool. This is like a basic stepstool, only in the shape of a "U" so that your baby can make a clear exit without crashing into a block of wood. They're sort of expensive — about $100-$250 — so unless you are planning several of these births and you're absolutely sure you're going to want to squat/sit for the final act, it may make more sense to borrow or rent one. (Don't think that you absolutely need a stool to give birth while squatting; there are other ways you can be supported in a squat position.)

Positive visuals. This will be different for every person. What gives you a calming effect? Perhaps a photograph of a blooming rose helps you to visualize your cervix opening. Maybe your wedding picture reminds you that you and your partner are in this together. Figure out what works for you, and start using the visual you choose to practice relaxation ahead of time. Then, when it's needed, the visual will be able to quickly take you back to that calm place.

Tell everyone to leave.

If you were having a home birth, the only people present would be you, your partner, your doula (more on doulas in Chapter 5's *Why your doula is more important than your husband*), your midwife, and perhaps her assistant. In a hospital birth, the list of people coming in and out of your room during the labor and delivery experience may include: you, your partner, your doula, your midwife, a nurse or two, a resident, a fellow, a medical student, a nursing aide, an orderly, the OB on call, and the group of family members and friends you called who are anxiously waiting for your news in the waiting room. That sounds like a private-event-turned-freak-show-circus nightmare if I ever heard one.

Part of the natural birth experience you are going for involves a quiet, calm atmosphere, with only super supportive people near. It's hard to go inside yourself and find your deepest focus and strength when there is a party of people watching you and chit-chatting with each other over vending machine snacks three feet away.

So tell everyone to leave. Just because you might be giving birth at a teaching hospital doesn't mean every Joe Schmo who got into med school gets to see your hoo-ha. Put a sign on the door that kindly reads something along these lines:

> *Inside this door is a laboring mother-to-be who has requested a quiet room. We appreciate the only guests be necessary medical personnel. Thank you for your cooperation.*

Make sure you tell your nurse about the sign. Perhaps she will ward off any potential offenders before they break and enter.

What you just learned

- Choosing your hospital and care provider is the single most important decision you will make about this birth.

- Not all hospitals or practices are created equal and it's never too late to switch to a different one that will give you a better chance at having your best birth.

- Ask lots of questions about policies and different scenarios before you decide to go with a particular care provider or practice. Know who the care provider's back-ups will be and if they have the same philosophy.

- Just because you're in a hospital doesn't mean it has to feel that way. Make it an environment that makes you comfortable and gives you the best opportunity to achieve the birth you want.

CHAPTER 4

It's easier than writing a term paper and much more important (your birth plan)

"Once you set your mind to it, it's your only option. I never even considered an epidural, even though I was in a lot of pain and didn't know exactly how I'd get through it. My thought was that the only way to stop the pain was to have the baby, so one way or another, the baby was coming out."—Emily Lancaster, who birthed naturally. She spent a lot of time laboring in the hospital shower, and her husband had the good sense to bring his bathing suit so he could hang, too.

If you've chosen your care provider and place of birth thoughtfully, the birth plan, or "birth preferences" as some prefer to call it, becomes less and less necessary. If your care provider and place of birth are completely in line with your desires for your experience, then you may not need one at all. This is likely true for someone having a home or birth center birth.

If you are having a hospital birth, even if you've carefully selected the mellowest midwife and the most holistic hospital with the lowest C-section rate in the country, it will serve you well to have a birth plan written out, if only so you become really clear about what you want. Additionally, in a hospital, there are many people taking care of you — not just that awesome midwife you picked out nine months ago and with whom you are now best friends. What if your midwife is out of town or otherwise unavailable? Even if another midwife backs her up, you'll want to make sure she has the same ideas about natural birth. You will have a nurse, and maybe two or three, depending how long your labor lasts. If it's a teaching hospital, you may have a resident come in at some point. If you don't want his less-experienced fingers giving you a cervical check (or anybody's fingers, regardless of experience), a birth plan is the place to indicate that wish.

So why do birth plans have a bad rap? Hospital workers see a lot of patients come through the L&D unit. They may even see a fair share of birth plans. They also see a lot of women who say they are going to hold out on an epidural, only to request it when they are three centimeters dilated. They see a lot of emergencies arise during labor and birth, and women who end up having life-saving C-sections. They are not inherently bad people. They just don't want to see your dreams squashed on that birthing bed, or sucked out of your vagina, via a vacuum-assisted delivery.

So it's important while writing your birth plan to keep in mind the people who will be reading — and hopefully following — it. Here are some tips:

1. Keep it short. It should under no circumstances be longer than one page.
2. Bullet points or list format make it easier to read.
3. Divide it into sections: preferences during labor, preferences during birth, and preferences for baby.
4. Use friendly words, like "we prefer" and "please." Remember that this is a wish list. Be kind to the people of whom you are making requests.
5. For procedures you absolutely do not wish to have, use the words: "I do not consent to…"; hospitals are more likely to pay attention to this type of legal phrase. You may also include this language in baby-care procedures, such as routine at-birth vaccinations or circumcision.
6. For procedures that you obviously prefer to avoid but would be willing to accept in an emergency, use this phrase: "I wish to avoid [insert intervention here, or just use 'all medical inventions'] unless in a life-threatening situation or requested by us. If a medical intervention is necessary, we would like to be calmly presented with our options with our doula and midwife, as well as 15 minutes to privately discuss the best way to proceed." True emergencies where time is of the essence and brief moments of decision-making will

make the difference between life and death are rare. When they do occur, they won't bother asking you; they'll just wheel you into surgery. You almost always have the luxury of 15 minutes to discuss. During those 15 minutes of discussion, you should be asking the care provider:

a. What are the advantages and disadvantages of the intervention you're suggesting?

b. What are some alternatives to this intervention?

c. Can we hold off on the intervention for now and reevaluate in an hour (or two or three…)?

Now you know the tone your birth plan should take. Here are the items you might want to cover:

1. Your labor and birthing technique (Bradley Method, HypnoBirthing, etc.)

2. Your wishes regarding:

   a. Environment (quiet, dimmed lights)

   b. Vaginal exams (as few as possible, or even none)

   c. No artificial deadlines (allow birth to proceed at its own pace)

   d. Freedom of movement (the fact that you want it)

   e. Medical interventions (that fact that you don't want them)

   f. Preferences in the event of a C-section (family-centered, gentle birth; skin-to-skin with partner)

3. Learn what procedures are routine at your hospital for your baby (usually Hepatitis B vaccine, vitamin K shot, and antibiotic eye ointment). Do your own research to determine if you want to agree to these procedures, or skip them. Remember, you are your baby's parent; you get to make all the rules regarding his care. Heavy stuff, I know! You wanted to be parents, remember? Include your desires in the "preferences for baby" section.

4. Also in the baby section, include your plans to feed the baby. You may wish to add that you would prefer that pacifiers not be given to your baby. Of course, this point is moot if the baby is always with you in your room, but it never hurts to indicate it in case of a NICU

stay or even a brief visit to the nursery for whatever reason.

What you just learned

- A birth plan should almost be superfluous if your care providers are completely on board with your desires; however, it's still a good idea to clearly state your intentions.
- You learned this one in kindergarten: Be nice.
- Include things that you want to take place and things that you don't want to take place.

Chapter 5

"I want an epidural"
(Getting through the pain)

"Stay away from negative people. I would ignore people who would tell me, 'Yeah, right, you're not going to be able to do it.' Don't watch reality labor and delivery shows; it will make you a nervous Nellie. Prepare for a natural birth — it's different from preparing for a different kind of birth."—Amanda Favreau, who birthed naturally after encouragement from her own mother who was an L&D nurse for many years and saw a few too many elective C-sections for her liking. She says that during transition, which was the worst part for her, she was complaining and asking for meds. Her husband made everyone leave the room so he could tell her "That's not what we want to do; we want to do this naturally," and he really got her refocused.

"If I didn't have the doula, I would not have done it; my husband would not have known what to say or do. [At one point,] I was asking anyone who came in the room for pain medicine. I even asked the guy emptying the trash."—Laurie Mazelin, who birthed naturally and confidently with the mindset that pregnancy is not a disability. She says she didn't need people holding doors for her while she was pregnant; she was actually

*stronger while in that state. Ultimately, she was glad
no one listened to her about the drugs (especially the
janitor).*

Yes, it's true. Despite everything I learned and researched over the course of
my pregnancies, despite how truly committed I was to my natural birth plan
that I distributed to everyone at the hospital, despite the fact that I would
love natural birth so much that I would go on to write this book, if you had
been in my delivery room during either of my labors, you would have heard
"I want an epidural" come out of my mouth.

Your partner, your hero

As it was, you were not in those rooms with me. My husband was. You know
what he said?

"No, you don't."

"No, seriously, I really do," I pleaded with him. "I changed my mind."

I have heard the idea of picking a safe word that you and your husband agree
that you will say only at a point of complete desperation, and that when you
say it, it means you mean business. It means you are allowed to cave to the
drugs.

I'm really glad we hadn't implemented this idea. If we had, I surely would
have shouted our safe word from the rooftop of the hospital. I would have
chanted it while dancing a jig around the L&D floor as I looked for the anesthesiologist.

I'm not saying this to panic you. Your plan for a natural birth is not in jeopardy of falling apart at the seams just because even this crazy birthy lady
showed signs of weakness. I'm saying this because I want to prepare you
for what you're going to be up against. Unless you have a really quick labor
(sorry, but unlikely for a first-time mom), or you have an unusually high
tolerance for pain, there is a really good chance that, in a hospital setting
especially, because you know it's available, you may decide at a certain point

that you can no longer stand the physical pressure of that little human being trying to get out of your giant womb, and you may say or think you want an epidural.

A lot of women say they are more scared of the epidural needle than they are of the pain of childbirth. I think these women say this when they are in the early stage of labor, and contractions are completely manageable. Hell, yeah, I'd take a couple menstrual-like cramps over a foot-long needle in my back! But once you are in more active labor, namely the transition phase, if you are still medication-free at that point, my guess is you will be running though the hospital halls, looking for the medicine man, begging him to stick that needle in your back.

I tell you this to make one very important point: **If you want a natural birth, your partner must be as committed to it as you are** (and perhaps even more so).

In defense of all husbands, partners and boyfriends who did not dare take the path that mine did, and actually listened to their laboring wives when they sought out pain relief, I can see why they do it. It's really hard to watch anyone in pain, but to watch the woman that you love crying and wailing, and know that it's pretty much all your fault that she's in this predicament, and that the only thing you can possibly do to help her is to agree to call the nurse and get her a freaking epidural, well, it's completely understandable.

When I was pregnant with my second child, I said a funny thing to my doula during a pre-birth meeting.

"I have a couple friends who have had really fast second labors. And I have been doing so much reading, yoga, and breathing practice. I really hope my labor is a little longer than theirs so I can really put everything I've learned and practiced to good use, and, you know, enjoy it."

"I'm going to make a note of that, and remind you in the delivery room," she said with a chuckle.

Thank goodness she didn't bring that up while I was pushing my little babutchkala out of my va-jay-jay, because in those moments — the same ones where I was requesting medication to take me out of my misery — I would have said that I had been wrong; that I wasn't enjoying it. That I didn't care about all the hours I spent in prenatal yoga classes or reading my own personal birthing affirmation statement each morning when I woke up. That all the time I filled sitting in a squat position to strengthen my quads and stretch out my pelvis could be for naught and I was fine with that.

But you know what? The amount of time it took for my husband to catch that baby and place her in my arms is how long it took to completely change my mind on that one. As a matter of fact, I enjoyed every single second of those extremely challenging moments leading up to the birth of my child. And I promise that you will, too.

I'm not saying I wouldn't have appreciated the entrance of my children without the accompanying discomfort, but rising up to the challenge of giving birth naturally made the experience that much more momentous.

So, how exactly do you get through it? Read on, my prego friend. Read on.

It hurts like hell. But with good reason.

Before we talk about dealing with the pain, it's really important that you understand why women experience pain during labor. And it's not because Eve took a bite from a damn apple, as the Bible will lead us to believe.

To begin with, mammals undergo physical discomfort at the onset of labor to let mom know that labor is beginning. The sensations are simply telling you, "You're about to have your baby. Find a safe place and get comfortable."

If you are an animal in the wild, you might find a quiet, secluded area, away from potential predators and chaos so that you can labor and birth in peace. It's actually quite common for mammals (this includes us) to begin spontaneous labor in the middle of the night or in the wee hours of morning. It's not by accident, either. Melatonin — the hormone that causes sleep[32] — works with oxytocin — the hormone that brings on contractions[33] — to

---

[32] What is melatonin: http://www.webmd.com/sleep-disorders/tc/melatonin-overview

[33] What is oxytocin: http://www.webmd.com/baby/tc/oxytocin-topic-overview

produce a synergy that promotes contractions forceful enough to do the hard work necessary for childbirth.[34]

If you are a natural birthing mama, you might call your partner and your doula and tell them both to head on over so you have your support peeps in place. You will probably pack your hospital bag if it's not in the trunk of your car already. And, like any mammal, you should set yourself up in a quiet and peaceful spot so that you can labor and birth with a semblance of tranquility. At first, this could be your bedroom or living room. Eventually, this will be your hospital room with the lights dimmed and only your support team in attendance. Even if it's not the middle of the night, you can mimic those conditions (dark, relaxed environment) in order to trick your brain into creating more of the melatonin hormone.

If there were no physical sign to let moms know that labor was starting, people would be birthing babies everywhere! You could be driving to work all la-ti-da and BAM! Out comes your baby on the driver's seat of your new minivan. You could be browsing the racks for some post-maternity clothes and BAM! Little junior is on the floor in The Loft dressing room. You could be enjoying some fro yo on one of those cool-looking-yet-oh-so-uncomfortable yogurt stools and BAM! Your own personal Little Me is knee deep in cookies 'n cream. And while the thought of having the baby so easily does sound sort of appealing, I'm sure you agree that it's best for this little bundle of joy to enter the world with a little less outside-world grime and with a little more notice.

Pain is also imperative during labor to serve an important physiological purpose. Unlike the pain you feel if you stub your toe or break your arm, the pain you feel in labor isn't because something is wrong. It is to encourage you to do the hard work necessary to complete the job of birthing your baby.

So what does that mean exactly? When you are having a contraction, your body's natural response is likely to move around. You might bend over, squat, do a few hip circles, or sway back and forth while holding onto your husband like you're at your first boy-girl dance. You aren't doing this to rec-

---

[34] A study on how melatonin works with oxytocin to promote contractions necessary for childbirth: http://jcem.endojournals.org/content/94/2/421.abstract

reate your puppy love romance. Your innate reaction of moving your body is actually facilitating your labor. Your movement during labor is also your natural way of coping with pain and making yourself more comfortable. Achieving small bouts of comfort will allow you to prepare for and tolerate the next contraction. Roll with it.

Some women may feel more comfortable coping with contractions by curling up and lying still. That's okay, too (though no one should stay in a single place indefinitely throughout labor). The important thing to remember is to listen to your body; if you do what feels best for you, it's probably exactly what your labor needs.

Luckily, your body is working with you on this crazy journey. All the intense sensations you're feeling are triggering your body to produce endorphins. These hormones will trick your brain into thinking the pain isn't so bad. Pretty cool, right?

The key to experiencing the joys of endorphins is that they only come on through contractions that your body produces on its own. This means that the contractions you experience when you are induced — the ones that are even more intense than naturally occurring ones and therefore harder to get through — these don't yield the pain-reducing hormones. Just another reason to let your baby choose his birthday.

Why your doula is more important than your husband

So now you know why you experience pain during labor; you just need to figure out a way to live through it. Enter THE DOULA.

If you're not familiar with the term, a doula, in its Greek origin, literally means "woman who serves." Who else would you expect to smile, say encouraging words to you, and bring you your every request while you're being a total bitch?

In the modern-day definition, a birth doula is a labor coach or assistant. You might tell me that your husband is your labor coach. False! He is your husband. Sure, he'll try to coach you. Kind of like how I might try to coach an NFL team. I've heard of football, but that doesn't qualify me to tell professionals how to play. Your husband has heard of a placenta (though he may still be a little confused about its function). That doesn't mean he is capable of leading you to the point of delivering yours.

Your doula and husband will become great friends in L&D, and they do share some jobs. Here is a list of some things either one might do:

- Rub your feet
- Fluff your pillows
- Bring you ice chips or snacks
- Tell you you're doing a great job

And here is a list of some things your husband has no idea about that your doula will do without thinking:

- Remind you to get up and pee
- Encourage you to move around, even when you say you don't want to
- Suggest alternative positions for labor or pushing
- Propose ideas for naturally inducing labor, if necessary
- Tell you to stop curling your toes during contractions, as this will tense up your pelvic muscles, too
- Allow your husband to eat and pee without the guilt of leaving you alone and unsupported
- Apply pressure to your back or hips appropriately to help you cope with each contraction
- Talk you through any decisions that need to be made throughout the duration, while supporting whatever choice you come to
- Coach you to push with your bottom muscles instead of your facial ones
- Remind you to smile and relax your jaw as this will encourage your cervix to relax
- Take photos if you request her to (including baby-coming-out-of-vag shots you won't show anyone, as well as the more tasteful very first family portraits)
- Record the whole event on paper since you and hubby won't remember any details

As you can see, your husband is necessary during birth because he's the dad and it was his sperm and all, but your doula is an actual essential member of your birth team who will get you from Point Pregnant through Point Some-one-Please-Kill-Me, and finally to Point I-Have-A-Cute-Stinkin'-Baby.

It's important to note that a doula is a non-medical support person. She is not there to tell you that you don't need a C-section or that your baby is in distress. She is not a midwife or a doctor. But she does know a thing or two about this birth stuff, and has certainly seen it in the flesh more often than you have. She can help to explain what is happening if you or your partner are confused, and she can guide you when you are debating your options. She is not there to communicate to your care provider what decision you and your partner make. She should always support whatever you choose. She is not there to pass judgment if you end up choosing an epidural or other interventions.

Some hospitals employ their own doulas, and for a fee or sometimes for free, you can have one attend your birth. While I applaud hospitals for rec-ognizing the doula's value, this isn't my preference. For starters, you won't meet your doula until you arrive at the hospital. And if you have a long labor, she might go home in the middle of it — just as you became comfort-able with her and got into a groove — and be replaced by a new one on a new shift. They both might be great at what they do, but it's really beneficial to have the same support person throughout the ordeal. You're not going to switch husbands halfway through, and you don't want to switch doulas either.

I am also not a fan of the hospital doula because, at the end of the day, she works for the hospital, which means she is not working for you. She answers to nurses and midwives and doctors, and she might not be as inclined as someone who you had hired privately to let you know when something doesn't seem kosher. Hopefully, you've chosen your care provider carefully and therefore you won't have to worry about an unnecessary C-section being suggested just because you aren't progressing fast enough. But even if you've done everything right, maybe your thoughtfully selected midwife or OB isn't on call on the night your little one decides to come, and you're stuck with a not-so-patient scalpel-happy doc. In this scenario, you want a doula who is on your side; one who will tell you honestly (and privately) that she isn't convinced you're ready for that step. Then you can make a fully informed decision about how to proceed.

A privately hired doula is my first choice. Find one that is certified through DONA International (www.dona.org), The International Childbirth Education Association (www.icea.org) or Childbirth and Postpartum Professional Association (www.cappa.net). Or ask around in the natural birth community, and you're sure to find a few local to you.

A privately hired doula usually costs anywhere between $400 and $2,000 (depending where you live), but some offer payment on a sliding scale; that is, you pay whatever you can afford. These women are passionate about helping women in birth, and although they are making a living this way, they are not in it for the money. When you think about it, even the most expensive ones, charging $2,000, are making very little per hour.

Your doula will typically meet with you once or twice while you are pregnant so you can discuss your birth goals and preferences. She will help you write your birth preference sheet (see Chapter 4). She will be available to you via phone and email for support in the days and weeks leading up to the big day. And when that day comes, she will be by your side from the moment you say you need her until after baby has his first successful nursing session. In case you haven't talked with anyone who has already been through this labor business, that event can take upward of 24 hours, sometimes longer. A doula's services usually also include a post-partum visit. So we are talking about maybe 30 hours total of work (and much of that is physical labor). That's about $66 per hour for the most expensive doula you can find. For a $500 doula, that's only $16 per hour. You probably pay your cleaning lady and your grass-cutting guy at least that much. You pay your manicurist, your hair stylist and your eyebrow wax chick even more. Soon you will pay a babysitter $50 so you can go spend $100 on a haircut.

The $600 that I paid my doula was the best money I ever spent. She gave me a form to submit to my insurance company for reimbursement, but as expected, doulas were not covered on my plan. Maybe they are on yours. You can write an appeal letter if they are not. Explain that you forwent an expensive epidural solely because of this doula who cost a measly few hundred bucks.

And that's not just by chance. Research shows that doulas significantly reduce your chances of using an epidural and of having a C-section.[35]

Why you should stop watching Birth TV and find a natural birth community

You've been watching "A Baby Story," "One Born Every Minute," "16 and Pregnant" or some other completely awful overdramatized bun-in-the-oven show ever since you took your first ovulation-kit temperature. Don't deny it. It happens to the best of us. They reel you in with the commercials of the upcoming episodes. *Will she end up with an emergency C-section? Will the baby daddy make it to the delivery room in time? Will the baby survive? Will the producers go to any lengths to present birth in the most theatrical and dangerous light?* I don't know about the first few answers because I stopped watching long ago, but the answer to that last one is a big fat pregnant yes.

From my standpoint, it would be completely entertaining to watch a completely uneventful normal birth, i.e. one where nothing goes terribly wrong and in the end you just get an elated mother and a pudgy little baby. Type "natural birth" into YouTube and you'll get to see a few of these — likely home birth — movies, though not in a neatly edited 30-minute format.

But I guess focus groups for television series determined that most people aren't like me, because it would appear that the only way to get ratings for a TV show featuring pregnant women is to weigh them down, not only with the heaviness of their swollen bellies, but also with the burden of the possibility of disaster at every point leading up to the birth. From gestational diabetes and high blood pressure to breech position and plummeting fetal heart rates, these shows will go to the ends of the earth to show how unsafe giving birth can be.

And I will admit that the act of giving birth can very well turn to tragedy. In a small percentage of cases, true emergencies arise, which would make for some great television (but a really scary situation in real life). But the

---

[35] More on the link between doulas and reduced rates of epidural and C-sections: http://ajph.aphapublications.org/doi/abs/10.2105/AJPH.2012.301201 and http://www2.cfpc. ca/local/user/files/%7B7E3888C2-49D4-4769-BB72-5FE433B9DE73%7D/Middle%20class%20 doula.pdf

rest of the time, things go fairly according to plan, or at least without major catastrophe striking.

Even if you've steered clear of shows specifically about L&D, you've certainly watched a regular sitcom or drama every now and then, and probably a few movies that happen to fit a new baby into the storyline. In fact, for the last 20 or 30 years (depending how old you are), you have been watching Hollywood's version of birth, and it's just not accurate. Women screaming and cursing at their husbands, extended families and friends walking into chaos-filled delivery rooms right as the baby is crowning, mother-to-be rushing to the hospital immediately after her water breaks as if the baby is about to drop out on the New York City street if she doesn't hail the very next taxi that drives by.

Many of these scenarios are ridiculous, and on an intellectual level, you know that. But over time, because of the repeated exposure to this preposterousness, your brain has been trained to fear birth. I'll repeat that one: **You have been trained to fear birth.** You weren't born with a natural anxiety over this very ordinary occurrence. It has been bestowed upon you, compliments of the western society in which we live.

I've got good news for you though: You can retrain yourself, not only to be unafraid of the process of birth, but also to be excited for it! (Keep reading, I'm being serious.) Remember earlier you read that I told my doula I hoped my labor didn't go by too fast because I wanted to enjoy it? I didn't say that because I'm a little crazy (though that's debatable); I said it because it was true. I had done so much retraining of my brain surrounding the topic of birth that I convinced myself that it would be an occasion to revel in.

How to retrain your brain to be fired up for the big day

The transformation from thinking that your body will surely split in two if you go through with this baby's exit, into thinking that the emergence of your baby into the outside world will be the best event you ever trained for isn't instantaneous. It takes more than a day, than a week, than a month (I hope you are less than eight months pregnant while reading this). Just as with any life-changing habit, it happens gradually over time, with practice.

The **first step** is to stop watching all the negative crap on TV (as detailed above). **Step two** is to stop talking birth with your mainstream friends. This is a bit of a toughie. You like your friends. They like you. And you're pregnant. And everyone likes to tell a pregnant gal her own birth story, however joyful or dreadful it may be.

Your mainstream friends had their babies in the hospital, attended by an OB, hooked up to a bunch of machines, many of them on an operating table. They will regale you with tales of their stalled labors ("I just couldn't get past five centimeters!"), their broken bodies ("There's no way that 9-pounder would have fit through these hips!"), and their horrid fits of pain ("I asked for the epidural to be waiting for me when I got to the hospital!").

So how do you benefit from hearing these accounts? I guess it makes for entertaining conversation over brunch. Beyond that, it adds no value to your pregnant experience. In fact, it detracts from it. Hear enough of those stories and you will start to believe that you'll be just like them. You'll start to doubt your ability as a woman in labor. You'll throw in the towel before you even have one contraction. The others did. So why not you?

Because you know better, that's why. To borrow a line from Maya Angelou, "When you know better, you do better." So man up, and tell your circle of friends that you appreciate them wanting to share their precious moments with you, but that you'd rather hear about them after you've experienced your own. It's also appropriate to let these nay-sayers know that your baby can hear them!

Step three: surround yourself with proud members of the natural birth community. To do so physically, you should sign up for a natural birth class. There are so many choices out there (HypnoBirthing, Brio Birth, The Bradley Method, Hypnobabies, Birth Boot Camp…the list goes on). Do a little research and decide what's right for you. You may make your selection based on philosophy, location of class, number of sessions, schedule, cost, or recommendation from someone. I chose HypnoBirthing the first time around, and Yoga Birth with my second (the version of Yoga Birth in which I participated is only available in Baltimore).

Many people asked me why I bothered with a class at all since I was a seasoned mother the second time around. I had already earned my natural birthing stripes. Surely I could do it again, right? Deep down, I knew that I could. But I was just one pregnant gal among many of my friends who were expecting their second babies as well. All of them had previously given birth with an epidural and were planning to do so again. In fact, an epidural was the only element in their birth plans, and although my friends love me, I think they secretly chuckled when the topic of my birth plan came up during our weekly playgroup with our toddlers. And you know what? That was fine. I am friends with these girls for a lot of reasons, but a shared view on natural birth is not one of them. If I was to be on the receiving end of any positive birth vibes, I was going to have to look somewhere outside my usual circle of friends.

In addition to a birth class, you can find support in the natural birth community in other ways. Even pre-birth meetings with your doula can perform this important function, as your doula can be a resource for you to learn about other places you can find support. Some natural baby stores hold get-togethers for pregnant women to network (and you can also use the time to pick out a sling and some cloth diapers, if you're into that). Some states and cities have a birth network group that meets monthly to discuss various topics.

Prenatal yoga was a personal favorite of mine; it gave me time to concentrate solely on my pregnancy (hard not to when the instructor is saying things like, "Breathe love into your baby") and it was a natural draw for other natural birth planners like myself. In one class I took, we went around the room before the yoga practice started for introductions. Each pregnant student said her name and where she was planning her birth, and if she had any questions or thoughts for the group. It was a nice way for some new and some veteran moms to comingle and share ideas and answers. If your yoga class doesn't officially do a meet-and-greet, casually introduce yourself before class begins, and invite a couple girls out for coffee after. (When I was pregnant with my first baby, I met a good friend exactly this way, though I have to give her the credit for the bold invitation.)

Instead of or in addition to finding a place to talk birth in person, you may want to reach out online for moral support. There are probably hundreds or thousands of natural-birth online communities out there, so do a little Google search and find ones that feel right to you. A few of my favorites are:

- tellmeagoodbirthstory.com /
  www.facebook.com / Tellmeagoodbirthstory
- www.mamabirth.blogspot.com / www.facebook.com / mamabirth
- www.banned-from-baby-showers.blogspot.com /
  www.facebook.com / bannedfrombabyshowers
- www.birthwithoutfearblog.com /
  www.facebook.com / birthwithoutfear
- www.facebook.com / pages / Giving-Birth-A-Fighting-
  Chance / 211385132257720
- empoweredbirth.typepad.com

Just seeing positive birth articles and stories show up in your newsfeed on Facebook can be a great subliminal reminder that birth is a normal event, and nothing to be afraid of. Depending how comfortable you are with blogs and social media, you may find yourself commenting on an article or in a conversation with a fellow mom-to-be. And now you have a new friend (and a free place to stay in another part of the country / world).

When everyone thinks you're nuts

Did someone say crazy? Yes, I did. Once you are uterus-deep in natural birth reading material and breathing techniques, you'll find yourself sharing your discoveries with anyone who will listen. This is me, a total natural birthing freak, telling you that you may wish to censor yourself just a tad when it comes to womb-speak.

I'm not saying you shouldn't be proud of your decision to birth your baby the way nature intended. I'm only warning you that unless you live on Ina May's Farm, there is a whole crowd of people around you who are not big supporters. (And if you don't know who Ina May is, a treat is in store for you! Ina May Gaskin is a respected midwife, author and activist. She is the founder of the Farm Midwifery Center in Tennessee, also know as "The Farm," which is noted for its low intervention rates and high successful outcomes. Learn more about her at www.inamay.com and pick up a copy of one of her books, *Ina May's Guide to Childbirth*.)

If you're opting for a home or birth center location, you'll have people scaring you about not having elements in place for an emergency. Even if your chosen setting is the mainstream-accepted hospital, people will have plenty of opinions for you. "You're using a midwife? Not a doctor? Is she even medically trained?" Your response, "Yes, actually she is trained specifically for attending *normal* births, not like doctors who, sadly, are often taught to treat all births like emergencies waiting to happen."

Even more educated people around you may be unfamiliar with some of the plans you have. "What's a doula? Is that like a midwife?" If your relatives, friends or coworkers have legitimate questions such as this one, and are interested in hearing an answer and learning more about your birth preparation, I encourage you to inform them about whatever aspects they seem fascinated by, but leave out the rest. Many people aren't ready to hear about concepts and practices that may at first seem unconventional to them.

A good strategy for helping those around you understand your perspective is to find common ground first. "Yeah, I definitely wanted to give birth in a hospital for the comfort of having emergency staff and tools right there, but I am choosing to use a midwife instead of a doctor so that the interventions would be kept at bay unless they become necessary." If you instead jumped right into why immediate cord clamping is so barbaric and how you plan to encapsulate your placenta for consumption, you will lose your audience right off the bat.

Another rule of thumb that took me longer to adopt was don't-ask-don't-tell. You'll surely be so psyched for your natural birth that you're going to want to tell everyone who tries to pat your belly in an elevator, but experience has taught me that it's best to save it for those who ask about your plans.

Perhaps you have a meddlesome mother-in-law, judgmental friend, or nosy sister who has made it quite clear that she thinks you're doing this all wrong. Don't fret. Chances are you think she did it all wrong. Let her know it's okay for you to have differing opinions, and you hope she thinks so, too. Tell her that if she's interested in having a receptive conversation, you're happy to explain to her how you came to your decisions. Once she learns about the thought and research that you've put into everything, she'll at least respect your choices, if not approve of them.

Be your own cheerleader

People probably already think you're off your rocker, what with your far out plans to give birth without drugs and perhaps with your pickles and ice-cream craving pairings. You may as well go with it.

Talking to yourself — specifically with affirmations and positive messages about your plans — will get you in the right mindset to achieve your goal. This will be helpful in all goals that you set in life, not just natural birth. Do you think marathon finishers look in the mirror each morning and say, "I think I might run a marathon. Maybe. If I feel like it. If I have time to train. If the weather is good."?

Hell, no. They gear up in ridiculously expensive running attire that promises to wick the sweat away from their bodies while keeping them warm in crazy cold temperatures that no one in their right minds would go outside in, and they run mile after mile while chanting to themselves, "I will run this marathon because I can and because I am awesome."

Maybe the above scenario isn't how everyone does it, but it's how I finished my marathon. True story: My sister and longtime running partner called me up on New Year's Day of 2008 and said, "We are running a marathon on March 29. Start training."

So I told everyone I knew that I was preparing to run a marathon. I knew I would be much more likely to go through with something knowing I'd have to answer to a hundred people if I didn't. And then the thought never occurred to me to not go through with it.

Even when I realized that January through March is a seriously cold time of the year on the east coast, and that I didn't enjoy running when I couldn't feel my fingers. Even when I invited a bunch of people to come cheer me on at the finish line and I was met with a disappointingly small amount of enthusiasm for a group of people who are supposedly my greatest support-ers. Even when I was at mile 22, and I looked to be running in a slow-mo-tion replay to anyone who might be watching. Throughout my 12 weeks of preparation, and 4 hours, 58 minutes, and 4 seconds of actual marathon time, it NEVER crossed my mind to give up.

And as someone who has both run a marathon and given birth naturally, I am qualified to tell you, *that* is the key.

If you have decided that you do not want an epidural, then remove that option from your brain. Yes, of course, you're giving birth at the hospital, so, technically speaking, it will still be an option. *But not for you.* You've just made up your mind.

You and I are friends, right? We've been together for at least a handful of chapters so far, so I feel like I know you. And I know that even though you seem really committed to natural birth at this point, there is like a teeny tiny half a percent of you that is still a little bit scared. *What if the pain is so bad that I can't take it? If I think my vagina will implode, or if I am in labor for more than 24 hours, or if my doctor suggests it, I reserve the right to change my mind and get the drugs.* Sound like any particular little voice you know?

I know you're tentative because, if this is your first baby, or your first vaginal birth, you are just afraid of what you don't know. I totally get it. It's really hard to prepare for something that you have only heard about. But I'm your friend, remember? And I'm here to tell you: YOU CAN DO IT. So stop with your what ifs and start with your affirmations.

Affirmations are just words. They are just statements that you make to yourself on a regular basis. Writing them down and saying them aloud are really powerful tools in making them happen. When words are written and spoken, they get outside your head and they become alive.

> *I will birth my full-term baby in a calm and positive environment, through a natural, mother-focused process, free of interventions.*

This was my official affirmation when preparing for the birth of my daughter. I wrote it on a little piece of paper with a line drawing of a pregnant woman (very Zen looking) in my natural childbirth class, and I kept it in my bathroom next to my toothpaste. Every time I brushed my teeth, I read it. Let's break the statement down, and while I do this, think about what's important to you so you can form your own statement.

> *"I will birth my full-term baby..."*

My first baby was premature, which was something I had never learned about or worried about, or even thought about the possibility at all. While pre-term birth is not the norm, it's more common than I knew (more than half a million each year in the United States[36]). I don't think it's something you need to lose sleep over; just something that you need to be aware of. Since I had already gone through a pregnancy that ended too soon, I was sure to be more specific when talking to the affirmation gods about what I wanted.

"...in a calm and positive environment..."

I was about to give birth in a hospital, not at a spa, though the latter was more the mood I was going for. When I think of hospitals, I think of frantic emergency rooms and hysterical patients on Grey's Anatomy. I think of needles and tests and bad news and worse food. But I didn't want my head to be in that place when I was preparing to meet my baby. *Calm* and *positive* were the terms I came up with to describe what I did want. I envisioned an upbeat, yet relaxed nurse telling me I was doing a great job.

"...through a natural, mother-focused process..."

Natural was the main event here, so I knew that word had to be in my statement. Many times, hospitals produce doctor-centered births — think scheduled C-sections and women in labor, ready to push but waiting for their doctors to arrive to "deliver" the babies. That's not what I had in mind. *Mother-focused* meant that it was all about *me*. How was *I* feeling? What position felt best for *me*? When did *I* feel the urge to push? Who did *I* want to catch my baby? I also included the word *process* to remind me that birth isn't instant. It took a long time to cook this baby inside me, and it was going to take however long it needed to take for it to come out. I didn't want to be on any timeline but my own and my baby's.

"...free of interventions."

Just me and my awesomeness. Nothing else, thank you very much.

So you should be totally inspired now. Take a few minutes, discuss it with your partner, and determine all the pieces you want to include in your affir-

---

[36] More on premature birth: http://www.marchofdimes.com/baby/premature_indepth.html

mation. Then write it down, many times if you are an over-achiever, and say it aloud at least daily from here on out. Tape it to your bathroom mirror or put it on the fridge. Rewrite it or move it around to new places every couple weeks so it doesn't become wallpaper that you don't notice anymore. This is your birth mantra. Say it like you mean it, and it will be so.

Remember, no one ever ran a marathon without *believing* they could do it.

What you just learned

- Birth is hard. But pain is not just a mean trick by Mother Nature. It actually plays an important role in the process.
- Invest in a doula. You are statistically more likely to achieve your natural birth goals with her there.
- Surround yourself with positive people and stories. Erase everything on your DVR. Ignore nay-sayers.
- Convince yourself that this birth will be amazing, and then it will be.

CHAPTER 6

What to expect when you're expecting this natural birth

"When it's at the worst it will be, it's intense, but it's for a short period. Just when you're about to give up is when you're almost there. If you've made it that far, you shouldn't give up."—Anne, who birthed naturally, and so quickly that she didn't use any of the birthing goodies (lavender, snacks, music) she had packed in her suitcase. She says the best part of having a natural birth was that it was the best thing she could do for her daughter. She says it "makes me feel a closer bond to her. And it makes me feel empowered as a woman... in a spiritual sense too. Nothing in my life will ever compare to that again."

"Someone told me early on — when you're in that pain and you think you can't take anymore and you're about to ask for help, the baby is almost there. Just push through it! This helped me get through. Educate yourself and know what your options are. People rely on doctors way too much — read as much as you can."
—Monica Pascatore, who birthed naturally two times. During the first experience, she was in and out of a self-induced relaxation trance for about five hours, just waking up briefly during contractions. They actually

had to wake her up to tell her it was time to push! Her second child came so quickly, she didn't have time to get herself into trance mode.

So you have all your hopes and dreams and a birth plan in place. You are saying your birth mantra every time you're at a red light. Now what?

Be patient like Cookie Monster

This is what I tell my kids whenever they ask questions like, "Are we there yet?" or "Is it my turn yet?" It started when they were babies and I read them a book where Cookie Monster has to wait for cookies to come out of the oven. You could learn a lot from that book.

When you're nine months pregnant and you're feeling glowy, confident, and huge, well, you wait. For contractions to begin, for your membranes to rupture, for your mucus plug to come out, for your cervix to ripen and open and thin, for the biggest poop of your life…all of these things are signs that labor is near or beginning.

What you're probably still wondering is: Once one or more of those things happen, when should you get this show on the road and go to the hospital? And the answer is as follows:

When you have been laboring at home for a while and your contractions have really picked up, that means it's time…

…to stay at home a little longer.

When your water breaks and you're dripping clear fluids all over your leather recliner for a few hours, that means it's time…

…to stay at home just a smidge longer.

When you are sure that the baby has dropped so low that you can feel the head coming out of your vagina, that means it's time…

...to get a mirror and see if that's actually the case, but if not, to stay at home for an itty bitty bit longer.

The bottom line is this: Once you get to the hospital, the game changes. Your labor actually changes. Maybe you were progressing nicely at home, but the change of environment, especially if it's not an optimal one, can put the brakes on your labor pattern. This is actually nature's way of protecting a laboring mother. If she feels at all unsafe, her body is able to essentially turn her labor off, because it would be dangerous for any mammal to give birth, for instance, with a predator nearby. And while you may not be afraid of a bear eating your baby, your body will shut things down if it senses any kind of fear in the laboring mother.

Even if you are going to the best hospital and the sweetest midwife is there waiting for you, the event of going to the hospital too early will still alter your experience. Remember, hospitals are businesses, and while they may not turn over beds as hurriedly as fast food joints clear your table, they still don't have endless time to let you labor in peace.

This doesn't mean you shouldn't be in touch with your midwife or OB once you know labor has begun. It's fine to check in with her via a phone call every few hours to give an update and so that she can sense where you are in labor. Chances are that if you can hold a conversation, you're still in the early stages and you have plenty of time, especially if you live close to the hospital.

You can also use your doula as a guide for when to hit the road. While your hospital midwife won't visit you at home, your doula will be there soon after you ask her to come. And although she isn't medically trained and therefore can't do a cervical check or anything of the sort, she can evaluate your demeanor and how you're handling contractions. She has seen a bunch more births than you have, so she is a fair judge of how you're doing and when it's a good time to get going.

An oft-referenced measure of hospital-go time is the 4-1-1 rule. That is, that you are having contractions every *four* minutes, lasting *one* minute each, for *one* hour. Try not go to the hospital until you've reached this milestone, because you are probably not that far along yet (and download a contraction app for your phone to keep track for you). It's worth noting that there are times when a woman could have contractions that are further apart but that last longer, and she could be in active labor. The best advice is to listen to your body, and check in with your doula or midwife. Either of these helpful ladies will be able to guestimate your progress by talking to you on the phone.

If your water breaks and you're not in labor

If your membranes rupture before you are actually in labor, it's called PROM: premature rupture of membranes (if you are before your 37th week, it's called PPROM: *preterm* premature rupture of membranes). If this happens, you should call your care provider. There are a few circumstances that indicate you should head over to the hospital right away, regardless of your labor pattern.

- If you tested positive for Group B Strep, a bacterial infection that you'll test for around your 36-week appointment. You'll need to be given antibiotics during labor to prevent passing the infection on to your baby. [37]

- If meconium is present. Meconium is your dear little unborn baby's first poop. If your baby poops in utero, your amniotic fluid will be greenish, yellowish, or brownish when your water breaks. It's more likely to happen in post-dates (past 40 weeks) babies because their guts are more mature. Meconium in the womb is bad news if your baby decides to inhale it. [38]

- If you are not full-term. Without amniotic fluid, the baby's umbilical cord could get squeezed between the baby and the wall of the uterus, and could even drop out of the vagina ahead of the baby (prolapsed cord). [39]

- If your baby is breech. Without the baby's largest body part — the

---

[37] More on Group B Strep:
http://americanpregnancy.org/pregnancycomplications/groupbstrepinfection.html

[38] More on Meconium Aspiration Syndrome:
http://www.nlm.nih.gov/medlineplus/ency/article/001596.htm

[39] More on prolapsed cord:
http://www.healthline.com/health/pregnancy/premature-rupture-membranes

head — down by your cervix, the risk of cord prolapse is greater.[40]

You really want to be in active labor when you get to the hospital, so hope-fully you can get to that stage at home. Here are some natural ways to help your labor along while you're at home passing time.

- Take a long walk. Or seven long walks.
- Jog up some stairs (carefully, you have a baby in there!). Try doing two at a time.
- Play with your nipples. The official term here is nipple stimulation. Use your own fingers, someone else's fingers or a breast pump. Have fun with it.
- Find acupressure points that are supposed to stimulate labor. There are some in the foot region, around the big toe and the ankle. If you don't feel up to Googling this for more specific instructions, just get a pedicure, or make a stat appointment with an acupuncturist.
- Eat food that gives you the runs. For some people, this might be some-thing spicy, or fried, or dairy. The idea behind this is that forcing your bowels to cleanse themselves can trick your body into thinking it's in labor, since your body will naturally cleanse its own bowels before labor starts. There are recipes available online that claim to work.
- With permission from your midwife, try a homeopathic tablet that induces labor.
- If you are brave and unafraid of massive poops, try castor oil. Some say drinking this nasty stuff will encourage your baby to come out; others say it merely assists your next 10 bowel movements to come out all at once. Don't say I didn't warn you. Ask your care provider what she thinks and what appropriate dosing should be.

Of course, your best course of action may be a preventive one — try avoiding the circumstance of your membranes rupturing before your baby is ready to arrive. Talk to your care provider about specific nutrition guidelines you can follow to strengthen your amniotic sac (ask about vitamin C, zinc and protein intake).

---

[40] More on breech position:
http://www.nlm.nih.gov/medlineplus/ency/patientinstructions/000623.htm and more on all kinds of fetal positioning: http://spinningbabies.com

Stages of labor: A numbers game

When you get to the hospital, they will do a cervical check to measure your progress. This is a pretty standard ritual of admittance, and I'm sure you're curious to see where you are in the process. If your water hasn't yet broken, and you're three or fewer centimeters dilated, they may not want to admit you. As the natural birthing mama that you are, you *don't want* to be admitted at this point. You are still only in early labor. (If your membranes have ruptured and you go to the hospital, you will be admitted immediately, even if you're not dilated at all.)

If you have made the misstep of going to the hospital before it's really time, I encourage you to go back home. I know, I know, you've been laboring all day, and it is starting to hurt really badly, and you just want this baby to come out. But being at the hospital is not going to make that happen any faster, barring medical interventions (which is precisely what we're trying to avoid, remember? I know you're pregnant and your mind has gone to mush, but try to keep up!).

As long as you haven't travelled a great distance to get to the hospital, your best bet is to make like Tom Petty and turn that car around. Get your pregnant ass back home and labor it out there. Alternatively, you can find a quiet area of the hospital to walk around. If it's nice weather, perhaps there is a garden area or a large fountain that doesn't get much foot traffic and just whispers serenity.

If you are dilated enough to be admitted, congratulations! You have completed the early phase of labor. Welcome to the "active" phase. As its name implies, this stage is a lively one. Gone are the long breaks between contractions. Gone are the mini semi-hypnotic naps while your partner rubs your feet. If you are in this stage, your body is doing the hard work of labor and you will know it. Even so, every hour or two, someone might come into your room and want to stick something up there to see "where you are." My advice: Tell them you're confident that you're progressing steadily and that you wish to skip this one. Here's why.

If they check you and you're not dilating at what has become the (arbitrary) expected speed — about one centimeter per hour[41] — not only will some care providers become impatient and potentially suggest augmentation, but you, yourself might get a little discouraged as well. After all, you are doing all this work and you want some dilation to show for it!

But your cervix may not have received the handbook that says how much it's supposed to open in any given time period. And you know what? That's okay. Because your cervix probably knows how to do its job just fine, even without that handbook.

Cervixes are funny things. They can take all day to dilate one centimeter, and then they can stretch four or five centimeters in less than an hour. And just depending on when you randomly check yours, who's to say that you're not about to have one of those really quick and effective bouts of progress? So pass on the cervical checks as much as you can. They are really unnecessary. You'll dilate whether you know you are dilating or not.

If you're not convinced, let me tell you a little story of my own personal experience with a cervical check. Here are my internal thoughts during my second labor:

> It's 11 p.m. I've been on the Pitocin drip for three hours (for my full birth story and why I had Pitocin, read *Liv Alexandra, born April 28, 2011* in Chapter 10 at the end of the book). I'm breathing slash moaning through some heavy contractions. The pain is beginning to get to the unbearable level, which I recognize might mean I am nearly fully dilated. Yes, I remember these exact sensations occurring just before the birth of my first child. I am, for sure, 10 centimeters dilated. I haven't had a cervical check since I arrived at the hospital seven hours ago and was only one centimeter, but surely, I am ready to push now.
>
> "Get the midwife in here! I need to be checked right now!" I say.
>
> As I grunt through the uncomfortable intrusion, I eagerly ask, "Well? Am I 10?"

---

[41] More on how quickly mothers "should" dilate: http://www.scienceandsensibility.org/?p=1439

"No, you're not 10," the midwife says.

And I'm guessing that if I were eight or nine, she probably would have said so instead of her ambiguous answer. So I decide that I don't want to know. That I can't know. Because if I know that I have progressed so little since I got here, and I indeed have to labor through this for more than another 15 minutes, I'll die. Or at least I'll get an epidural. Yes! An epidural! I forgot all about that option! (Go back and read Chapter 5's *Your partner, your hero* on how I didn't get an epidural.)

I labor on for two and a half more hours — the hardest work I've ever done to date — and my baby girl is born at 2:07 a.m. after 20 minutes of pushing. I ask my midwife how dilated I was during that 11 p.m. check. She tells me four-and-a-half.

Four-and-a-half freakin' centimeters! I'm glad I had the wherewithal to realize that I didn't need to know that number at that time. It would have finished me. I didn't know that in the span of less than three hours, I'd expand five and a half more. And that's my point. You just don't know how your cervix will behave on the big day. In this story, no one was dissatisfied with my progress besides myself, but if I had it to do over again, I would have waited longer to get that check, and hopefully would have avoided the discouraging news (or lack of news, which I found discouraging).

Once you reach about eight centimeters (whether you know it or not), you have moved on to the latter part of active labor, called transition. The good news is you are almost finished — only two centimeters to go. The bad news is, this one is a doozy. Transition is intense. I will try my best, but no words can prepare you for the spectrum of pain that is possible during that timeframe, when the baby is beginning to descend down the birth canal.

You know what a menstrual cramp feels like? That's sort of the sensation you'll feel when you first start having contractions. You'll think you have a stomachache, and then after you realize your stomachache is coming regularly every 5 minutes or so, you'll come to grips that you're in labor. "These are contractions?" you'll say so sweet-and-innocently. "I can totally handle natural birth!"

Then the active phase begins and you have fewer breaks between contractions and you're really using all the methods you've read about and practiced to focus and get through them. "This isn't sooooo bad," you'll say. "I can get through this."

When transition hits, you'll try to get out the following words (if you can find the time between back-to-back contractions): "Forget it. I decided I don't want a baby. Let's go home." This is quite common for women in transition. When you think it's quitting time, you'll know the end is near (and don't worry; you'll decide that you really do want your baby, after all). Your labor support team is extremely important during this phase. You'll need them to help you get through each contraction individually. Don't worry about what's coming next; focus on making it past the contraction you are having right now. This technique will get you to the end of this road and onto pushing.

Just know ahead of time that transition will be challenging, but really rewarding when it's over. In fact, women often experience a short break after becoming fully dilated before having the urge to start pushing. Enjoy it!

Squatting: It's not just for killer quads (movement and positions during labor)

Now that you've stopped watching fake birth in the movies and "real" birth on TLC, the idea that everyone gives birth while lying flat on her back should be but a faint memory for you. Start watching videos of natural birth on YouTube, and you'll see that almost no one births this way unless forced by an epidural or encouraged by a care provider.

You'll want to move around as much as you can during labor. This movement will not only help you cope with labor pains, but it will also do the very important work of bringing your baby down into the right position. Remember, gravity is your friend. If you're lying flat on your back, gravity helps baby do nothing; if you're standing up, sitting upright, or on your knees, gravity is encouraging baby to move down.

So, what does this movement look like? Whatever feels good for you. Pacing around the room, holding onto your husband in a middle school slow dance stance, and sitting or bouncing on a birth ball are all good places to start.

Many women find the toilet to be a great place to labor because the natural inclination while sitting on the crapper is to release your pelvic floor muscles. If you've been tensing up your pelvis, just sitting on the commode for a few contractions should help to relax that region. On the flip side, if your contractions are already pretty powerful, you may not like this location as it may increase the intensity too much too soon.

You can also go to the bathroom to actually pee or for a really lame field trip of sorts. Just the movement of walking back and forth to a new, albeit relatively close location, and going from sitting to standing up can not only pass the time, but also help with the progress of labor.

Hydrotherapy — a fancy word for anything you do with water — is also a fantastic tool for labor and is often called "nature's epidural." If you're lucky enough to be at a hospital with a birthing tub, fill that bad boy up and get in! Don't forget to bring your partner's swim suit so he can climb in, too, and massage your back while you're in there without it being weird for others in the room (as it might be if he were naked).

You'll want to be in steady and active labor when you get in; soaking up all that relaxation might actually slow your labor down and we don't want that to happen. Whether you're tubbing at home or in the hospital, get the okay from your care provider first, as high blood pressure or a fever would be reasons to stay away from water immersion.

If you don't have the luxury of the big tub, a shower can work as well. The water running down your body can help calm and relax you. You won't be tricked into thinking you're on a spa vacation, but it sure beats the hospital bed.

Even hospitals that do provide birthing tubs won't always allow you to actually give birth in them (so call them labor tubs, okay?) so you have to be armed with effective and comfortable birthing positions.

Anything that keeps you vertical is working with gravity, and therefore is making it easier for the baby to come down. You can use a birthing stool, which is like a horseshoe-shaped stool so that the baby has an open spot to come out. You can kneel on the bed while leaning onto the back of the bed (where the pillow goes). You can squat on the bed while holding onto a squat bar (check to see if your hospital supplies this). You can squat on the floor while holding onto a chair, a birth ball, or your partner. You can go doggy-style on all fours, either on the floor or on the bed. You can sit upright on the bed while holding your knees toward you.

Believe it or not, there are even more possibilities, and your doula or midwife will have suggestions for you based on your particulars of labor and the position of your baby. Find physical support wherever you need it through your partner, your doula, a ball, a chair, a bar, or pillows. And in whatever position, always work with your contractions; not against them.

Get ready to make your own *National Geographic* soundtrack

If you have had the pleasure of moving a human being through your pelvis, then you already know that silence, soft whispers, and sweet nothings are not on the playlist.

Here's what is: primal, loud, embarrassing, potentially sex-like noises that you didn't think your voice was capable of making.

Go ahead, decide right now, "No way I'm going to be one of those loud, laboring women! I'll have my baby with a few 'hee-hee-who's'; thank you very much." Only one problem: it's sort of not up for discussion.

I said it was primal because it's not a choice you make as a sophisticated, manicured, high-heel-wearing species. The doctor doesn't instruct you to do it or not to do it. These sounds will just emerge from your mouth as naturally as your baby will emerge from your vagina, albeit with much less effort. And just like the pain that essentially helps your labor progress, these noises play an important role, too.

Breathing with low-pitched sounds can help a laboring woman to relax and her cervix to open. Asking your birth team to join in with you isn't out of the question, and may even help more.[42]

Moaning is also an instinctual way of coping with pain or discomfort, so embrace it. That's one more option for you in your arsenal of tools to avoid the epidural.

If your baby is sunny-side up

The real term is called occiput posterior fetal position, or OP for short. It means that if you are lying down on your back, the baby is on her way out facing the ceiling. She is ideally supposed to come out more or less facing the floor — that is, her head is meant to more easily glide through your pelvis in that position with her chin tucked on her way down the birth canal.

Having an OP baby can mean that your labor lasts longer and that you experience your contractions more in your back than in your belly, as the bony part of the baby's head is pushing against your pelvis during contractions. It can mean you will have harder work to do than someone whose baby is in an optimal position. It can mean that your labor will be stalled and you will need to change positions more often. It can mean that you will forever be saying to your child, "I knew you were going to be trouble from the moment you were facing the wrong way in that delivery room!"

Babies end up in less than ideal positions due to maternal habits during pregnancy like slouching on the couch, too much time spent driving, not enough time spent walking, and poor nutrition. Staying in only one position during labor can also be to blame, or sometimes just plain bad luck, so don't beat yourself up over it.

An experienced midwife or doula will have tricks up her sleeve for encouraging the baby to turn during your labor or even as late as during her exit. But even if those methods aren't successful, know that an OP baby can be born vaginally and even without operative (vacuum or forceps) assistance.

---

[42] More on sound during labor: http://www.firstbreathathome.com/sound.html

If you think your baby may not be in the optimal position, visit www.spinningbabies.com for a lot of information on that topic.

Why don't you try squeezing something the size of a watermelon out of an opening the size of a lemon and see how hot YOU look?

I heard Kirstie Alley deliver that line in *Look Who's Talking* when I was 8 years old, and it really stuck. I knew babies came out of vaginas, but I really didn't get just how that was possible. I also knew that my vagina opening wasn't as big as a lemon, as this really realistic movie suggested [insert sarcasm]. For years, I thought I was in trouble.

As it turns out, during all that hard work you do during labor, your vagina *does* open to the size of a lemon, and then through the pushing stage of labor, something the size of a watermelon *is* able to make its way out. Facilitating that process is both an art and a science.

The first thing to remember is to have patience. The baby doesn't come shooting out like you've been made to believe when a character gives birth during a 22-minute sitcom. Pushing can take anywhere from a few minutes (not likely during your first birth, sorry) to several hours. Try not to think in terms of "how much longer do I have to go" while you're experiencing it. Just know that with each passing minute and contraction, you are one minute and one contraction closer to the grand finale.

Tell your doula ahead of time that you'll want a mirror while you're pushing. You'll be too distracted at game time to remember, so she'll take care of requesting one for you. I remember being a little discouraged when I used the mirror during my first baby's birth. I felt like I was mustering up every last bit of effort I had inside me, and all I saw was a quarter-size bit of my baby's hairy head trying to come out. So let's try to mentally prepare for that picture. It will look like nothing is happening, but I assure you, progress is taking place.

You may also see in the mirror that during one big contraction and push, your lady parts open really big, and you're all, "I'm there! This baby is coming now!" And then three seconds later, the contraction is over, you relax, and your vag goes back to pocket-change status. Then you're all, "What the heck!? I'm moving in the wrong direction!" Rest assured. This opening-and-closing process is what you want to take place so that your hoo-ha goes back to its original size and location after this whole baby business is over. If you push too quickly, too hard, and without breaks in between to return your vagina to its regularly scheduled size, you are more likely to tear or sprout hemorrhoids.

Many women are under the impression that everyone either tears or is given an episiotomy; that one or the other is inevitable. And while I'm not saying that natural tears *never* happen, I am saying that not every woman tears, and that fewer people would if their care providers were more patient and respectful of the process.

Mother-led pushing means that you push only when you feel the urge to do so; not when a doctor yells "PUSH!" and a nurse counts to ten like some deranged preschool teacher beside you. Going along with this holding-your-breath-for-10-seconds idea can be called "purple pushing," and, as you might expect, you'll probably turn purple if you do it. You also might pop a blood vessel or two in your face (in case vaginal injury wasn't causing you enough worry). Purple pushing evolved for women who needed to be coached when it came to pushing — the ones with epidurals who couldn't feel the urge themselves. If you're not sure when to push, you can certainly ask your care provider if it's time, or if the sensation you're feeling means it's time. Pushing only when you feel the urge is a good defense for tear prevention.

Another tear-prevention method is called "laboring down." This term refers to the process by which you postpone pushing until the baby has made his way down most of the birth canal on his own. Although laboring down means you are just hanging out instead of doing the hard work that is pushing, it is probably harder to do than pushing, especially when you're not medicated, because sometimes you are resisting the urge to push.

It's sort of like when you first feel like you have to poop. If you go the moment you feel it coming on (let's compare that to the moment you become fully dilated), you'll have to do some pushing to get it out. But if you hold it in for a little while (let's compare that to resisting the urge to push), like if you were in a long line at a concert, then the minute your butt hits a toilet, BAM — poop is out with no work at all.

Laboring down can slightly increase the total time of your labor, but it's probably negligible, and might be worth the effort if it means an intact vagina. While you're not pushing, you'll just be letting your body do the work for you with the benefit of you not becoming exhausted. If you've heard of a mom spitting a baby out in just a couple of pushes (especially if she had an epidural), she didn't just win the baby-crowning lottery; she probably labored down.

Lots of lube works well too, and hopefully your midwife has a big bottle of the gooey stuff within reach so that she can slather it all over your precious baby's head each time he gets closer to the finish line. You may also ask her about doing perineal massage (slow stretching of the skin between your vagina and your butt — more on this in *Chapter 7: But I'm still afraid: Letting go of fear before labor*) while you push. But above all else, *patience*, on the part of everyone in that room, is your vagina's best friend. You'll thank me later.

What you just learned

- Patience is a virtue. Stay home as long as you possibly can before going to the hospital.
- Avoid cervical exams during labor to avoid discouragement. You will dilate whether or not you know it.
- Try all forms of natural induction before moving on to medical ones.
- Use squatting and other positions that feel good to you during labor and birth.
- Your vagina is elastic. It will stretch as big as it needs to. Seriously, it will.

CHAPTER 7

But I'm still afraid:
Letting go of fear before labor

*"I was so confident about birthing one baby, but was
scared when I learned it was two."—Alissa DeBernardo,
who birthed a singleton naturally and a couple years
later, after she got through the initial fear of two
babies coming at the same time, twins. She says the
most painful part of the whole twins experience was
when a nurse leaned over her so forcefully to sneak
a peek at the action, that she strained her back (the
second twin was being extracted by a medical resident,
breech-style, which is something medical staff don't get
to see often).*

At this point, you may still feel apprehensive about this whole birth business. Don't worry, you're not alone. It's totally understandable to be scared of the unknown. But it can also be dangerous to the process, so let's work on eliminating your fears surrounding birth before the big day.

How can being afraid of your own vagina be dangerous to the process? *Sphincters* are circular muscles that surround the opening of an organ (such as your bladder, rectum, cervix). They are called upon to empty themselves at appropriate times. These openings ordinarily remain closed but have the ability to open as widely as needed when necessary. Ina May Gaskin coined the term "Sphincter Law" to explain that sphincters work best in private, intimate settings; they don't respond well to commands like "Push!"; and they can suddenly close if their owner becomes scared.[43]

---

[43] Watch Ina May Gaskin discuss sphincters: http://www.youtube.com/watch?v=dCfSZn28FgM

Here's the deal. Your cervix is a sphincter. It typically "remain[s] closed" but has "the ability to open as widely as needed when necessary." That means it stays shut, but opens when it's time to have a baby. At least, that's what's supposed to happen. When you're afraid of birth, or even of baby-related topics, you can subconsciously get in your own way of your cervix opening. It's like your body is trying to do whatever it can to stop this kid from coming.

Past sexual abuse or any type of unresolved grief can play a part here as well. It's important to find a professional to talk with about these issues, not only for your own mental and emotional well-being, but also for the health of your pregnancy and baby.

Scared that birth will ruin your sex life forever? Nervous about the financial responsibility a little one will bring to your family? Anxious that your relationship with your husband will change when all your time is dedicated to feedings and diapers?

What better way to alleviate these worries than to change your mind and not have this baby after all? That is what your cervix is thinking. The only way around this is to remove those concerns beforehand.

Before you can remove them, you must identify them. They are different for each woman. You may have none on this list or you may have all of them. If there is a fear listed below that you haven't thought of yet, please, don't adopt any new ones! I only mention them so that I can help you be rid of them, not so you can develop additional birth phobias.

Pregnant women report on many reasons to be afraid, including, but of course not limited to the following:

Missing signs of labor

This is a reasonable fear in that you've never experienced labor so how are you to know when it's happening? But it is pretty unlikely that you would be able to ignore signs of labor for long enough that the entire thing takes place without you knowing it. And if you were so lucky that your labor is so painless, what's the worst that can happen? You give birth on your kitchen floor?

Great! Then you get to have the home birth you probably secretly wanted anyway but were too afraid to have.

Seriously, even if you miss the first few signs of labor, you will surely recognize it once you are in a strong pattern of contractions. If that doesn't convince you, perhaps you'll be one of the lucky women whose water bursts, and then the puddle you're standing in will confidently let you know what's going on. And, in the very worst-case scenario, if you have a labor that progresses really quickly and you truly miss all the opportunities to go to the hospital, then call 911 to get a quick ride to the hospital post-birth, and call your midwife to guide you and your partner through the experience over the phone.

If it makes you feel better, take some time now to research delivery-related information, like how to resuscitate a newborn if it were needed. But don't get too caught up in that; only 10 percent of babies need a little help breathing once they're born (and less than 1 percent need "extensive resuscitative measures") which means the large majority knows what to do on their own.[44] And don't worry about cutting the cord; it's likely best for baby if it stays attached until it stops pulsating on its own anyway, which would be the case by the time the ambulance your partner called when you both were freaking out arrives to check you both out.[45]

If you happen to have an accidental home birth, the most important piece of information you need is something you will do instinctively: just hold your naked baby close to your skin with a clean blanket thrown across to keep her warm. You will hopefully also get the chance to do this in the more likely event of your planned hospital birth.

Being forced to stay in bed during labor

If you are forced to stay in bed from the time you're admitted to the hospital, your labor will be disturbed, possibly slowed down or halted, and the interventions will likely begin. But if you've done your homework, you've

---

[44] More on neonatal resuscitation: http://pediatrics.aappublications.org/content/126/5/e1400.full

[45] More on delayed cord clamping: http://www.scienceandsensibility.org/?p=5730 and http://foxnews.com/health/2011/11/16/umbilical-cord-should-not-be-cut-for-3-minutes-study-says/

chosen a hospital and a care provider without such rigid rules, so you needn't worry.

To set your mind at ease, bring this question to your next appointment: Under what circumstances would I be forced to stay in bed during labor?

1. Just being in labor and admitted to the hospital
2. If my water breaks
3. If I need an IV for fluids, antibiotics or Pitocin

Hopefully, the answer is a big N-O for all counts. If the answer is yes, follow-up with a "But can I get up to use the bathroom? And can I just stay near the bed, but be upright, walking or sitting on a ball?" For reasons due to circumstances, I was confined to bed to some degree for both my labors. But the bathroom excuse was awesome; when you're that pregnant, you have to pee every 15 minutes anyway, so no one suspects you're trying to pull a fast one. With my second child, I wasn't bedridden at all; I just had to stay close enough to my Pitocin drip, which gave me about a three-foot radius to play with (plus potty breaks).

It's certainly not ideal, but it's not the end of the world either if you find yourself at a hospital where that is the law. So find out what the rules are where you'll be. And then stop worrying.

That the baby won't fit

If you're five feet and your husband is six-foot-seven, it doesn't mean your baby won't fit. If you normally wear a size zero and your mother-in-law has casually mentioned that your hubby was a 10-pounder, it doesn't mean your baby won't fit.

Nature typically doesn't make babies who aren't in perfect alignment with their mommies. So if you're a petite little peanut, and you're married to a Sumo wrestler, your baby will still end up at a reasonable size for your uterus and vagina.

The whole large-baby thing is an actual condition called macrosomia, but it's fairly uncommon, and often misdiagnosed. Unless you have gestational diabetes, excessive pregnancy weight gain, or are 44 weeks pregnant, chances are your baby is a normal size, even if a late-pregnancy sonogram shows he is "measuring big." Guess what? Sonograms that are done later in pregnancy (37 weeks or later) are actually less accurate than ones done earlier in the third trimester.[46]

Still afraid you might pop out a 3-month-size newborn? Think about this: A *mule* is the offspring of a *male donkey* and a *female horse*. This hybrid animal has historically been bred because of the combined traits that it inherits from its parents.

A *hinny*, on the other hand, is the offspring of a *female donkey* and a *male horse*. So it technically has the same genetic makeup as the mule — who remember, has a donkey dad and a horse mom — but in general, is much smaller in size. "Hinnies are smaller because donkeys are, for the most part, smaller than horses, and growth potential of equine offspring is influenced by the size of the dam's womb."[47]

Now, I'm no scientist, and perhaps I'm the first to make this analogy, but this makes perfect sense to me. A donkey's womb is smaller than a horse's, so a donkey mommy's baby will be smaller than a horse mommy's baby, regardless of whom the dad is. And if my womb is smaller than someone else's and therefore won't hold as much, then my baby will naturally be smaller (or at least small enough to fit).

Don't let a doctor tell you that your hips are too narrow to birth your baby either; what kind of cruel joke would Mother Nature be playing on us if she made women the wrong size to birth their own babies?

Tearing and then needing stitches

I admit this doesn't sound terribly pleasant, but it really isn't something you need to list on your catalog of fears. If you tear, you tear, and you'll get a few stitches. The end. Your vagina will go back to normal (or at least a new

---

[46] Here's a study on the "Prediction of Birth Weight by Ultrasound in the Third Trimester": http://journals.lww.com/greenjournal/Fulltext/2000/04000/Prediction_of_Birth_Weight_by_ Ultrasound_in_the.6.aspx

[47] More on hinnies: http://www.reference.com/browse/hinny

normal that you'll learn to love). In fact, the first time you have sex after birth, you'll feel like a virgin again, and your worries will not in any way be along the lines of how stretched out you are down there, but rather about how a penis ever fit up there to begin with.

The actual feeling of tearing isn't something to be afraid of either. There will be a lot going on in the moment, and you won't feel the sensation of tearing while you're concentrating on birthing your baby.

To prevent tearing, your care provider should guide you in slow-paced pushing, using lots of lubricant. You can also prepare for the big day yourself starting at about 34 weeks, when you and/or your partner can perform perineal massage for about 10 minutes daily. Perineal massage is when you or your partner gently massages and stretches the perineum — the area between your vagina and anus — to help prepare it for the stretching that will occur during birth. It isn't the fun foreplay it sort of sounds like, but it's probably better than tearing and sitting in sitz baths for 10 days after birth. Don't forget to use lubricant. According to one study, perineal massage decreases the risk for tears in first-time moms by about 10 percent.[48]

That I will poop during labor

Even if you're afraid to admit to this fear, we all know that you are scared shitless (or maybe full of shit?) that you will take an enormous crap on your delivery bed while pushing that rug rat out. One benefit to the epidural that I haven't mentioned thus far is that should you have the unfortunate experience of pooping in front of a room full of birth supporters, at least you won't feel it happening. But you'll probably smell it so you're not really protected anyway.

If you poop during the pushing phase, it is truly not a big deal. Doctors, midwives, and nurses see this happen ALL the time. No one will point at you and laugh (well, you might want to make your partner agree to that ahead of time, just in case he has a nasty sense of humor and a burning desire to sleep on the couch). Honestly, no one cares, including you. That's right: When it comes down to a few final pushes, you will be making promises

---

[48] More on perineal tearing: http://www.pregnancy.org/article/perineal-massage and http://www.scienceandsensibility.org/?p=5899

with the birth gods that you'll go back in time and poop at your senior prom if it means this baby will come out sooner.

That I will end up with a C-section

If you're giving birth in America, where the C-section rate was 32-33 percent in recent years, this fear is a valid one.

But look at you — you're doing your research, you're choosing your care provider carefully, you're reading this awesome book — you have nothing to be worried about! If you do end up with a C-section, you will feel confident that you medically needed one, in which case you will be grateful that you were in the hands of qualified doctors who helped bring your baby safely into the world. And there is nothing to feel guilty or shameful about that.

While I don't want you to plan for a C-section, or even be of the lackadaisical mindset, "I'll do whatever I need to for a healthy baby" (of course you will; is there any mother out there who feels otherwise?); I do want you to be prepared for one.

How do you prepare for a C-section without planning one? Simply include in your birth preferences a few lines about "in the event of a medically necessary C-section" how you still wish for a gentle birth experience:

- Immediate skin-to-skin contact (if not possible with the mother, then with the father)
- Delay newborn assessments
- Reduce family separation to a minimum

Women who have C-sections can still feel satisfied with their birth experiences, so long as their voices were heard and respected during the process. This will surely be the case for you if you chose a care provider you trust. It's okay to seek out support as you grieve for the birth experience you didn't get to have, even if the end result was a healthy baby.

That something will be wrong with the baby

This is a common fear, and one that might plague you throughout pregnancy. If you've had all the testing recommended by the American Congress of Obstetricians and Gynecologists, you can at least rule out many serious abnormalities that may worry you. As for the rest, just get used to the constant state of concern and responsibility; it's a huge part of parenting. Even if your baby comes out picture perfect, there are thousands of reasons you will worry about her physical health and emotional well-being before it's time for kindergarten.

I remember once before I had children, my mother-in-law told me she couldn't sleep because she was worried about some facet of my husband's life (maybe he had a cold or some other minor complaint). And I was like, "He's practically 30 years old, I'm pretty sure he can handle it." She said, "Just you wait. Have a baby and you'll never sleep again."

Whether or not you're a sound sleeper for the next 30-plus years, the point is that you will love your baby no matter what. Your baby is a part of you, and you are all he or she has in this world. You have the rest of your life to worry about this child; try to hold off on it for the sake of your birth experience.

That something (anything) will go wrong

Okay, calm down. Your pregnant brain is in overactive mode. Yes, things can go wrong during birth. But they usually don't. And you've been taking care of yourself. You're eating healthy foods, exercising safely, meditating daily, and going to all your prenatal appointments, smiling as you gain pound after pound after pound of pudgy mommy goodness. You are pouring love into your giant belly all the time. You are giving birth in a hospital that you have researched, where you know there are capable hands to take care of you and your baby. You're doing a great job at being this kid's mom already!

Don't get me wrong. While I want you to be positive, confident and hopeful, I also want you to be realistic. Minor setbacks happen that might steer you off your best laid out plans.

Maybe you'll be Group B Strep positive, and so you have to go to the hospital sooner than you'd like for antibiotics. Maybe your baby comes too early. Maybe you're 42 weeks and you're baby doesn't seem to be coming ever. Maybe you need an induction. Maybe your water breaks but you're not in labor. Maybe all the breathing and coping tricks you've practiced just aren't cutting it. Maybe your partner isn't as supportive of your choices as you'd like. Maybe your doula is on vacation and you can't reach her backup. Maybe your baby is breech and won't turn. Maybe your baby becomes distressed during labor. Maybe you need a C-section.

There are a thousand more maybes that might happen. Just know what your goals are, and try to stick to them as much as you can while being flexible for new developments along the way. You are stronger than any scenario that may be thrown at you.

What you just learned

- There's a lot to be scared of when it comes to birth.
- That first one was a trick to see if you were paying attention. Really, there's a lot you might be scared of, but not a lot you should be scared of. Work through your fears sooner rather than later.

CHAPTER 8
Whose baby is it anyway?

"My baby was born with severe tongue-tie and upper-lip-tie. I suspected a problem with her latch when she was born, so I sought out the advice of three pediatricians and three IBCLCs [International Board of Certified Lactation Consultants] to find a solution to all our nursing issues. I got a lot of terrible advice, mostly to just supplement with formula or to wait it out. I wanted so badly for my daughter to have the privilege and health benefits of exclusive breastfeeding, so I kept pushing."—Sarrah Yoder, who was finally able to exclusively breastfeed after much persistence and insistence to many pediatricians and finally an ENT that her daughter needed to have her lip-tie released. *"As a new mother, I quickly learned that my greatest role, next to protecting and nurturing my baby, is to be her best advocate."*

Now that you've squeezed that baby out, it's time to be his mom. Not just you-want-to-kiss-him-to-pieces kind of mom; like a real *mom*. I know it's scary, but this human being is depending on you to make all of his big decisions. At this point, those decisions might involve whether or not he wears a hat, but that is big stuff to a dude with no hair and no way to regulate his body temperature.

Sometimes when you give birth in a hospital, it takes a little longer to realize that the baby, who was most certainly yours when he inhabited your abdomen, still belongs to you now that he is earth-side. I don't mean that

103

you don't feel an immediate love connection with those chubby cheeks, but the enormity of becoming a parent can take a few days to register. Add into the mix the authoritative nature of doctors and the like in our culture, and you might be left unsure of what is in your control.

In short, everything about your baby falls under the category of what is in your and your partner's control.

I'm not encouraging you to be a crazy helicopter parent from the moment he starts breathing air; I just want you to know that you are in charge of your baby. For instance, the nurse might try to give your little guy a bath within his first hour of life, or while you get settled into the mother-baby room. That might be standard protocol and she's just doing her job, but that doesn't mean you shouldn't get to soak up your baby's first suds of cuteness in the tub yourself. Kindly let her know that you'd like to give the baby a bath yourself, maybe later that day or even the next day. There's really no rush to bathing a brand new baby. Sure, he comes out kind of gooey, but he didn't just roll around in the mud. The vernix covering his body actually contains various antimicrobial properties, protecting a newborn against a wide variety of infections. The white filmy stuff also happens to be highly moisturizing, and seriously, nobody likes dry skin.

The nurse may come in later during your stay for your baby's hearing test or blood draw (required by some states). Ask if these procedures can be performed in the room with you present. At 24 or 48 hours old, there isn't much that should separate a baby from his mama.

Always follow your gut when it comes to your child; you need to be his advocate

When my son was born at 34 weeks' gestation, he spent eight days in the NICU. The doctors and nurses there were wonderful, and I am so grateful that we were in a hospital with such a high level of neonatal care available, and even more grateful that my four-and-a-half pound bundle didn't need much of it, besides a heat lamp and some monitoring.

I think it was around day five or six of his stay when the doctor sat us down and told us that Dylan was progressing so nicely, and that he wasn't quite ready to go home yet, but that he had graduated from needing the intense care provided by the NICU. He was ready to move into the Pediatrics unit of the hospital. She said I'd be more comfortable there because I'd be allowed to stay in the hospital overnight (I was discharged as a patient on day three, and had been traveling back and forth to the hospital each day after sleeping at home). My husband and I were initially elated — our baby was almost ready to come home!

But in those first few days, I had come to feel almost at home in the NICU, and I was nervous about these unchartered waters they called Peds. So I asked if we could have a look at what Dylan's new digs would look like, and how it worked on that floor. On the NICU floor, I was used to having a swipe card (given only to NICU parents) that let me into the locked unit's waiting room, and then a NICU staff person had to personally let me or any other visitor into the actual space where all the babies bunked. A nurse was assigned to one, two or, at most, three babies (if they were all pretty healthy and didn't require too much attention), and she was sitting near them all the time, ready to swoop in if necessary.

On the Pediatrics floor, I learned that you just hopped off the elevator to the second floor to gain access, so pretty much anyone tall enough to reach the elevator buttons could roam the halls and poke their curious heads into your room. And while yes, I was allowed to stay overnight in Dylan's room, we'd be sharing that room with another child and possibly his mother, too. Dylan would be trading in the cozy glass bassinet that he had become accustomed to sleeping in for a harsh-looking metal crib, the baby equivalent of a jail cell, I thought. As soon as I saw one young toddler standing up all by his lonesome in his sad excuse for a bed, I burst into tears.

Granted, I was totally postpartum, a little sleep-deprived, and dealing with the emotions of having an unexpected premature baby in the Neonatal Intensive Care Unit. I wasn't exactly the picture of emotional stability. The nurse giving us the guided tour of the second floor gently moved us back to the NICU office, where I said I did not feel comfortable moving Dylan to Peds, and that I wanted him to stay in the NICU until he was ready to come home. She immediately agreed.

Later that day, I overheard the doctor giving the same your-baby-graduat-ed-the-NICU speech to a neighbor of Dylan's, and little Johnny was moved to Peds that night. It turns out there was a mom in labor, and they needed to clear out some space in the NICU for her preemie twins.

I tell you this story, not because I think I'm the best mom ever and Johnny's parents didn't give a rat's ass about him. I'm also not saying that Pediatrics is a bad place, and I'd be thankful for that unit I'm sure, if my children ever needed to pay a visit there. What I am telling you is mostly something I learned by watching Oprah (am I the only one whose life lessons all come from this source?). And that is that if something is not quite right, you first hear it as a whisper; and then a louder sign appears, until finally you are hit in the head with a brick telling you what you need to do. Don't wait to get knocked out by the brick — listen for the whisper if something isn't as it should be. If you feel a little uncomfortable, it is your intuition talking.

What's this kid gonna eat?

This isn't a book about why you should breastfeed, but chances are that if you're entertaining the idea of natural birth, you are intending to breast-feed, anyway. Good for you! As you know, breastfeeding begins at birth. So let's arm you with some tips for successful breastfeeding in the hospital, where your birth will take place. Replacing even one feeding with formula in the first few days of life can adversely affect all the effort you are putting into your early breastfeeding relationship, so you'll want to be prepared beforehand.

Come on, how can one measly bottle change your nursing relationship? Glad you asked. For starters, nipple confusion. This is where a breastfed baby tries a bottle, and then, the next time you offer him your breast, he forgets how it functions. When a baby latches onto and then sucks milk from a breast, the mechanics involved are much more complex than when he simply takes a rubber nipple between his lips and gravity allows the milk to drip into his mouth with hardly any effort on his part. When you introduce a bottle too early, the baby can become confused about which nipple he's getting, and apply bottle-drinking methods at the breast, which will hurt your nipple and inhibit the milk from coming out.[49]

---

[49] More on nipple confusion:
http://www.askdrsears.com/topics/breastfeeding/common-problems/nipple-confusion

You can imagine the cascade of effects that happen after that, but I'll play it out for you. Baby nurses at the breast just fine after birth. Baby gets a bottle or two while at the hospital. Once discharged, Baby forgets how to nurse at the breast, or gets lazy at having to work (read: suck) to get the milk out. Baby cries when nothing comes out. Mommy cries because the latch is incorrect and her nipples get sore. Mommy cries more when she doesn't know why Baby is crying and begins to be worried that Baby isn't getting any milk (which he isn't with the dreadful latch he's using). A well-meaning grandmother suggests just giving a bottle so that Mommy can relax and not be stressed that Baby is starving. Mommy is at her wit's end so she agrees. She spends the next 12 months exclusively pumping or supplementing with formula. She misses out on the close bond nursing mothers get, and she feels cheated out of a beautiful experience and relationship.

If you want to get all scientific about it, there's another reason to not introduce formula to your breastfed baby. Brand new babies have sterile gastrointestinal tracts. Babies who are exclusively breastfed have a more acidic gut environment, and naturally develop lots of good bacteria and not a lot of bad bacteria. Babies who are formula-fed have more bad bacteria, and therefore are at higher risk for illness. As soon as you initiate a formula diet for your baby, his "virgin gut" as they call it — a gut that's only ever had breast milk — is changed.[50]

At birth, your baby's stomach is teeny tiny. Like the size of a walnut. Seriously! He needs only the few drops of colostrum that are trickling out of your boobs (maybe even as you read this). He does not need a premade bottle of artificial milk. Your milk will come in around day four or five. And he will not only survive, but be totally satisfied with your colostrum until then.

There may be some dire circumstances that would require supplementing at this early stage, but those are rare. Ask the pediatrician if he thinks giving your baby a bottle of formula right now is completely *urgent* and *necessary*. He's likely to say that you could wait a bit longer to see if [baby pees, baby gains weight, etc.]. In the meantime, put that baby on your breast as often as you can to stimulate your milk to come in. Be sure to include a feeding

---

[50] More info on gut stuff:
http://dralexrinehart.com/nutrition-benefits/importance-of-breastfeeding-infant-gut-development
and http://www.thealphaparent.com/2011/07/virgin-gut-note-for-parents.html

preferences section on your birth plan. Hopefully, this will ensure that the topic of formula doesn't get broached unless medically necessary.

You may indeed want some rest while you're in the hospital. And while you can certainly get rest while keeping the baby with you at all times during your stay, you may wish to send the baby to the nursery so that you can sleep more soundly. If you do so, make it abundantly clear that you wish to be woken up as soon as the baby wakes up, whether or not he is crying, and that under no circumstances do you consent to a bottle (and maybe not even a pacifier, depending how you feel about that; some feel that early on, it's best for the baby to take care of all his sucking needs at the breast). It will be good for your milk production to feed the baby as often as possible.

Ask for the lactation consultant to come visit you every day that you are in the hospital, *even if there are no issues*, and breastfeeding seems to be as easy as giving candy to a baby. She will confirm that you're doing everything right and that the baby is getting the hang of this new skill. If you do have issues that develop or persist, continue seeing a certified IBCLC (International Board of Certified Lactation Consultants). Most breastfeeding challenges can be overcome as long as they are addressed early.

What you just learned

- This baby belongs to you. You make the calls, right or wrong, from here on out.
- Breastfeeding success can be shaped early on starting at the hospital. Get a solid start by feeding on demand and often, and by passing on the bottle at the hospital.

CHAPTER 9

Top 10 things
to take away from this book

So there you have it. Everything you need to know about birthing your baby naturally at the hospital. At this point, you should feel educated, empowered, excited, and completely enthused about the journey ahead of you.

If you're looking for the Cliff's Notes version or a cheat sheet you can carry around with you, here it is. If you want to achieve the natural birth you've been dreaming of in the safe space of the hospital, here's what you need to know, in abbreviated form.

1. Commit to natural birth. You are the only one who can make this happen.

2. Assemble a supportive birth team (i.e. get your partner on board and hire a doula).

3. Wisely choose your medical attendant and hospital. Pick someone you know you'll trust fully if things don't go exactly as planned. Be flexible if your plans need to change.

4. Retrain your brain to know birth is normal and not scary. Become excited for birth.

5. Set your intention. Write your birth plan and an affirmation statement. Read it and say it aloud often.

6. Identify your fears surrounding birth and let go of them. You don't need unresolved anxiety getting the way of your cervix opening on the big day.

7. Practice physical and mental relaxation. You need this during birth and you should be skilled at moving yourself into a relaxed state.

8. Immerse yourself into a like-minded natural birth community, both physically and online.

9. Exercise patience. You will need it when you're 10 months pregnant and waiting for labor to begin, and when you've been in labor for

10 hours and are one centimeter dilated. You're in this for the long haul.

10. Own it. This is the only chance you have to birth this baby. Do it the way you and nature intended! And enjoy it. Happy birthing!

CHAPTER 10

My own birth stories

This book is about you and your journey to prepare yourself for a natural and totally fulfilling birth experience. But in case you're wondering about the credentials of the person giving you all this information, here's the natural hoopla I went through to meet my own little ones. As you'll see, I did not always have the picture-perfect natural births I longed for, but I kept an open mind, made adjustments to my plan when necessary, and stuck to my guns on the parts most important to me. And guess what? I ended up with three empowering and awesome experiences that I wouldn't change for the world.

Dylan Jack, born April 29, 2009

When you're a childless couple, as you may know, you can have sex with your spouse whenever you want. As was the case on a random Monday at 6 a.m. before my husband and I got up for work. After we did the deed, I lay still in the bed for a few minutes until I knew I'd have to get up and begin my week. Suddenly, a gush of fluid was coming from between my legs. My husband shouted, "Stop peeing in the bed!" to which I desperately replied, "I'm trying!"

I ran to the bathroom to finish whatever was happening in the toilet, and was even able to catch some in a little Dixie cup for inspection. I noticed the liquid was a little bit pink-tinged. Nope, I had not peed in the bed. Indeed, my water broke.

I was 33 weeks and 6 days pregnant.

When you're not expecting to be in labor for another six weeks, you don't have your hospital bag packed. You don't have your dog sitter waiting for The Phone Call. What you do have is a frantic husband running around the bedroom throwing his clothes in a duffle, and a fairly large pregnant chick using your last sheet of computer paper to print off the birth plan to bring to the hospital.

I hadn't considered a premature labor during the entire eight months I was pregnant. They don't teach that to you in childbirth classes. They don't talk much about possible NICU stays or steroids they can give you to push your baby's lungs into high gear so he's ready to be born, even when he's not supposed to be.

But in all honesty, I wasn't that scared. I had taken HypnoBirthing classes (all but the last session, which was to take place that evening), and I had trained my brain to be very relaxed surrounding everything with this birth. Even though I knew it wasn't an ideal situation, I knew that a nearly 34-week-baby wasn't in grave danger, and that ultimately everything would be fine. Once we were admitted to the hospital, I was filled with adrenaline and excitement, knowing I'd be meeting my baby sooner rather than later.

However, I was a little concerned that my plan to give birth naturally was in jeopardy. I didn't know anything about pre-term labor or preemies. Was it safe for them to be born vaginally? Was a midwife allowed to attend the birth of a preemie, or did I now fall into the category of "high risk," requiring a doctor? I was told that while I was now considered a high-risk situation, my midwife could still attend the birth, and there would be a team of NICU nurses there to evaluate my baby when he was born.

I quickly learned that the 34-week mark was a milestone of sorts; that if your labor begins at that point, the hospital staff will not try to stop it; prior to 34 weeks, a laboring woman is typically given drugs to stop contractions. I was at 33 weeks and 6 days, but the high-risk obstetrician who consulted with my midwife on the case decided I was close enough, and it was okay to let me be. Other than the fact that my membranes had ruptured, I actually wasn't in labor at all — no contractions — so they were just going to wait for my labor to begin on its own.

I had heard that you couldn't hang out with your water broken for longer than 24 hours or else there was a risk for infection. What if my labor didn't start in the next 24 hours? I brought this up to the high-risk OB and she said the risk of my baby being born too early was of greater consequence than the risk of infection, and that we could monitor me to make sure I wasn't developing one. She also mentioned that they could induce me on Wednesday (two days later, once the steroids they gave me would have taken full effect to develop the baby's lungs) if I hadn't had the baby by then. I quickly agreed.

When the high-risk doctor exited the room, I was left with one of the midwives I'd been seeing during the last 14 weeks of my pregnancy (I had switched to a midwife practice at 20 weeks). She told me in a hushed tone that I did not have to be induced on Wednesday, and that if I wanted to stick to my plan of a natural birth, then to forget the induction. I could remain with my water broken and no baby for much longer, she assured me.

At that moment, I felt so happy that I had made the switch to the midwife practice. The high-risk OB on my case, who I just met that morning, certainly knew that I wouldn't be in danger if she didn't induce me on Wednesday. So why had she so casually said we would do just that? She didn't ask me if that was okay with me, or present it to me as one of several options. She simply heard my concern that I'd be at risk for infection (as had been drilled in my head from years of listening to other people's birth stories and cautionary tales from their own doctors) and gave me the quickest solution to address that concern. My midwife, on the other hand, knew my intentions, and gave me a few moments of her time to explain to me that I still had choices. Even though my situation had changed, I was still a player in this game, not a spectator.

Later that day, I met with the neonatologist from the NICU who told me that a baby born at 34 weeks gestation was required to stay in the NICU for a week at the very least, and that the baby's condition would dictate if that stay had to be longer. He said his concerns for the baby were underdeveloped lungs (which were being addressed with the steroids I was given already, assuming I could stay pregnant for another 48 hours for them to take effect), low birth weight, and the ability for the baby to keep his temperature warm enough. There were small chances that he'd have other, more serious problems, but we didn't need to worry about those for now.

Throughout Monday and Tuesday, I had contractions on and off. I was confined to the bed except for trips to the bathroom after a sonogram confirmed that the baby's head was in the right position and the cord was not in front of it. (When the cord comes out before the baby, it is called umbilical cord prolapse and is very dangerous; this is extremely rare but less so in the case of prematurely ruptured membranes.) I had a constant electronic fetal monitoring belt strapped to me, which was not only uncomfortable, but also really annoying when it would move off the exact right spot on my belly, which would send a nurse running to my room to see why they could no longer hear my baby's heart on the monitor at the nurses' station.

By Tuesday evening, the contractions had become regular enough that we called my doula and told her to come on over. We thought the baby must be on its way. But instead, some family members were on their way to visit me, and soon after their arrival, my contractions stopped once again. At the time, I hadn't thought about my parents and sisters as being sphincter inhibitors, but in hindsight, I'm fairly certain my body just didn't feel comfortable laboring in front of an audience. So it stopped.

My doula went home. I was moved to an antepartum room since I wasn't in labor and they needed the Labor & Delivery space for women in actual labor. The good news was that I was allowed to eat, finally. I had been on a diet of semi-clear liquids (which included apple juice, Italian ice, and chicken soup) since I arrived. Most hospitals will not allow laboring women to eat, and some stricter hospitals ban beverages other than water, too. Their rule didn't seem so bad until I had been in some form of labor for two days. A girl who's growing a human being gets hungry! So I had a bagel and cream cheese at 10 o'clock at night and then — whaddayaknow — my contractions came back. I told the nurses I wanted to be moved back to the Labor & Delivery part of the floor where I'd be more closely monitored by the nurses' station. Once we moved to L&D, I went to bed.

I slept well for a couple of hours and then in dribs and drabs from midnight to 2:45 a.m. on Wednesday morning as the contractions became more regular. At that point, I woke my husband from whatever sleep he may have been getting on an upright chair, and he asked me if he should call the doula. I felt badly about waking her in the middle of the night, especially since she had already been to the hospital the previous evening, just a few hours earlier. What if this was another false alarm? No, I told him, let's wait until a midwife checks me and we know this time it's for real.

Well, I guess the midwife was delivering someone else's baby or something because it took her 45 grueling minutes to come to my room and measure my cervix. When she finally made it, I told her I'd changed my mind and wanted the epidural. She told me it was too late; I was 9 centimeters dilated.

"Let's call the doula now," I said, since I was getting ready to push. She got there in time to be extremely helpful during pushing, but I wished I'd had the benefit of her presence at the start of those tough contractions. I'd know better for next time.

The midwife suggested I begin pushing by sitting on my knees and facing the back of the bed. Eventually I turned around in a regular seated position and pushed for a long time this way. The nurses brought in a mirror so I could watch my progress. I saw a quarter-sized patch of dark black hair creeping out of my vagina, and I was so excited to get it out of me. But every time the push was over, the quarter turned into a dime and then just a little black speck, and I didn't understand why, with all this work, I was going backwards. I didn't know at the time that slow-and-steady wins the birth race, and that this paced pushing was going to save my vagina from tearing.

After an hour and a half of this in-and-out business, my tiny baby popped out all in one push into the midwife's hands. He was placed on my chest right away, and I asked what this cute little bundle was while I held my son for the first time. My husband told me it was a boy.

I got to hold him for just a few minutes before he was taken across the room to be evaluated by the NICU nurses. I was elated with the time I got under the circumstances. Although nothing was of immediate concern, his gestation required he be taken to the NICU and monitored there. I was reunited with him a couple hours later and was allowed to visit him there as often as I liked throughout his eight-day stay.

I had achieved my first natural birth. It wasn't as I imagined it. It wasn't completely perfect. But it was exactly what I wanted nonetheless. I had rolled with the punches and became flexible to my plan as necessary. It was the proudest I'd ever felt. I rocked that natural birth high for weeks.

Dylan Jack Rauseo was born at 5:23 a.m. on April 29, 2009.

Liv Alexandra, born April 28, 2011

After having a preemie, my main goal was to carry this pregnancy to term. I learned that even though 40 weeks is what everyone knows to be the usual gestation for a human, 37 weeks is indeed considered full-term. And even if I only made it to 36 weeks this time, a NICU stay would not be required for this baby.

Because of my preterm ruptured membranes the last time around, I had been taking a shot of progesterone every week since about 20 weeks during this pregnancy. This wasn't a get-out-of-the-NICU-free card, but there was a chance it would help me carry the baby to term. A pregnant woman's body naturally produces progesterone, but the extra dose was supposed to aid in keeping me pregnant longer. And I think my husband enjoyed sticking a needle in my ass every Thursday night for months.

My final birth class — this time I took Yoga Birth — was on a Monday night when I was 36 weeks and 6 days pregnant. When I signed up for the course, I was afraid I'd have my baby before the session was over and I'd be wasting my money on only half the classes. But now I was out of the woods. I felt some extra pressure low down in my pelvis as I walked to the car, but just assumed it was the baby dropping some.

When I got home, I went to sleep and woke up several times to pee (as usual). At 3 a.m. I woke up again, but it seemed as if maybe I'd already started to pee when I ran to the bathroom. I wasn't 100 percent sure, but I thought my water broke. It wasn't the gush that I remembered with Dylan, so I wasn't positive. But then I started having mild, but regular contractions every 5 or 7 minutes, so I figured it was my water. And it continued to trickle out, so I was sure I couldn't still be peeing two hours later.

I rested for a couple hours during these contractions, and then they kind of stopped altogether, so I figured I would use the time to get myself ready for the birth. I packed my own hospital bag for this birth since, in my husband's frenzied hurry last time, all he managed to pack me was my pregnancy journal and Chapstick.

All day Tuesday, my contractions were sporadic. I only had one or two per hour after those initial couple of hours following my water breaking. I had my scheduled 37-week visit with my midwife that afternoon, so when I was there, she did a sterile speculum exam to confirm that my membranes were ruptured. She did not do a regular internal exam so as not to increase the risk of infection. She confirmed what we both already knew.

At that point it had been 12 hours since my waters had broken. She said her "official recommendation" was to go to the hospital, but that really it was up to me how long I took to get there; 6 hours, 12 hours… I felt really happy that my midwife (the same one who told me I didn't need to be induced with my first baby) clearly knew my birth intentions, and was respecting my desires to obtain a birth free of interventions. We both knew if I went to the hospital with a full-term pregnancy and ruptured membranes but no contractions, I'd immediately be put on a Pitocin drip.

So I spent the rest of the day trying to get my contractions going again. I took a long walk, used my breast pump for nipple stimulation, ate spicy Chinese food, walked up the stairs two at a time, did squats, and did acupressure on my big toe, above my ankle, and on the skin between my thumb and pointer finger. Some of these things did bring on a contraction or two, but nothing that stuck or that got my labor into any regular pattern. I tried distracting myself by doing my nails. Still nothing.

I went to sleep Tuesday night figuring my labor would start up while I was resting and I'd be ready to go to the hospital by morning. But I woke up at 3 a.m. after only a few contractions and decided that at the 24-hour mark, I needed to stop sleeping, be more proactive, and really get this labor started. So my husband and I climbed out of bed and started everything all over again. We walked around the neighborhood at 4 in the morning and were the first customers at Starbucks when it opened at 5. When I paid for my latte, the barista looked at my round belly and asked when I was due. I bet she was surprised to hear my answer: "My water broke yesterday. Thanks!"

I called the hospital around 6 a.m. and spoke to the midwife who was there at that time. She made me feel better about the situation saying that she felt comfortable with me staying home until I hit 36 hours with ruptured membranes, and that she really only felt that I needed to deliver the baby by 48 hours. I told her I was really worried about going to the hospital and getting Pitocin, and that it would surely ruin my plans for a drug-free birth. She told me she had birthed both of her own children with Pitocin and without an epidural. Until then, I had never heard of someone doing that. I truly hadn't thought it was possible. Now I had some hope.

She also suggested I try a homeopathic tablet to bring on labor. We killed some more time going to a couple different stores trying to find it (if your care provider recommends this; go straight to Whole Foods).

At 36 hours, it was 3 p.m. on Wednesday, and labor had completely stopped, no contractions at all. I was mentally ready to go to the hospital at that point, and even figured that I'd need augmentation eventually, but based on the conversation I'd had with the midwife in the morning, I thought that I still had time to bring on labor naturally in order to deliver by the 48-hour mark.

With my premature son, my water had been broken for a full 40 hours before I started active labor on my own; though in that situation, the hospital allowed me to stay pregnant with ruptured membranes for much longer with no questions asked, since the risk of infection was secondary to the risk of a preemie. But I was thinking that if my body worked that way the first time, maybe I just needed a full 40 hours this time to get started, and I really wanted to give it a chance.

So I called the hospital and spoke to another midwife. She was new to the practice and very inexperienced. She said she had talked with the OB on call at the hospital, and that I should definitely come in right away, and that they would start me on Pitocin immediately. I was devastated. Was she giving me this advice based only on what the OB said? I wanted an opinion from someone who knew me and my plan; not from a doctor who only saw me as a patient chart. I wished that another midwife was working so I could get a more experienced point of view.

I told her that I really wanted the chance to walk around some more, to try to get the labor started naturally. But I also really wanted to go to the hospital because I felt a strong desire to have the baby monitored so I could be reassured that everything was okay. I got a little emotional because I didn't know what I wanted more — to not have Pitocin right away, or to have the baby monitored. Right before we hung up, I'd said that I didn't know whether or not I'd be coming in right away given the circumstances. The midwife could tell I was upset when we got off the phone. She called me back a few minutes later to say that she really wanted me to come in to have the baby monitored, and that we'd evaluate my options once I was there. I felt a little better then; maybe my voice would be heard, and I wouldn't be forced into the Pitocin right away.

We went to the hospital at 4 p.m. (37 hours post-ruptured-membranes) and our doula met us there. As soon as I got to triage, I was put on the electronic fetal monitor and the contraction monitor, and lo and behold, my contractions started! They weren't strong, but they were regular. And the baby looked fine. The Labor & Delivery unit was really busy that night so the midwife just left us alone; she knew I wanted only to be monitored and to stay off the hospital radar for a while anyway.

At about 6:30 p.m. she came into my triage room. She said that she thought it was time to admit me and start Pitocin to augment my labor; the contractions I was having weren't strong enough yet to be considered active labor. The change of shift was about to happen at 7 p.m. so I asked if I could wait to talk to the next midwife. I knew that the next midwife coming in was the same one who'd examined me in the office the day before, the same one who I trusted so completely after my experience with her during my first labor.

As soon as the change of shift happened, the midwife was detained assisting in a C-section, so that bought me another hour or so. By the time she came to see me, it was 8:30 p.m., and by then, truth be told, I no longer minded the idea of Pitocin. I had reached the 41-hour mark, which was all I really wanted to do on my own without the intervention, and I still was not in active labor. And if this midwife said it was time for the intervention, I knew that it really was.

I started Pitocin at 8:30 p.m., and labor picked up right away. I was sure to tell them to give me the lowest dose possible, and to increase it at the minimum level (the nurse said they usually increase it by 2 units every half hour but only did it by 1 unit for me).

I asked the nurse if she had seen my birth preferences, and she said, in a not-so-reassuring tone, "Yeah, well, you're heading down a road you don't want to be going down." She was referring to the long duration my membranes had been ruptured, and similar scenarios she had seen in which this circumstance precipitated an infection and then a C-section. I got kind of upset about her negative attitude and obvious lack of support, but remembered that I had my midwife, my husband and my doula, and I could still do this naturally, even if the snarky nurse didn't think so.

For a couple of hours, the contractions picked up steadily and got longer and stronger. I just breathed through them, often hearing my Yoga Birth teacher's voice in my head: "I am aware of myself breathing in, I am aware of myself breathing out." This was the active stage of labor where I was serious and in a rhythm by myself. My husband and my doula were just hanging out in the room, taking the time to rest themselves or rub my feet. I was in my own world, solely focused on breathing and relaxing my body to encourage my cervix to open.

By 11 p.m., things had picked up quite a bit, and I started needing more help to get through each contraction. Even though I was hooked up to an IV for Pitocin and an antibiotic, and to the EFM and contraction monitor (required because of Pitocin), I still had about a three-foot radius of space that I could walk around. So I tried several positions at this point; lying on my side on the bed, sitting on the birth ball next to the bed, hands and knees on the bed, knees on the bed while hanging over the birth ball, and standing while my husband sat on the bed and supported me.

Eventually, the contractions seemed to be back-to-back with only short breaks in between. It reminded me of the hardest part of Dylan's birth right before the end, so I imagined I must be really close to fully dilated. I'd had only had one cervical check—upon being admitted to the hospital, and I was one to two centimeters at that point. I said I wanted to be checked again because I was sure I was close to 10.

The midwife checked me. "No, you're not 10."

"Please don't tell me I'm only 4," I begged her.

"No, you're more than 4." But her tone didn't sound reassuring, and I was terrified that I still had a long way to go. I asked her not to tell me what the number was so that I wouldn't be discouraged further. I asked if the Pitocin could be turned down a little because if I still had a ways to go, I couldn't bear the thought of the contractions I'd been having (or worse, ones that were stronger) for several more hours. They turned it down.

The next two hours were really challenging. I was extremely vocal to get through every contraction. Without a doubt, I could not have gotten through this period without the help of my husband and my doula. Again, I was switching positions often in attempt to find a comfortable one and, subconsciously, to help move the baby down and into an optimal position. My doula applied pressure to my hips during every contraction, which was really helpful physically, while my husband stood in front of me and let me squeeze his hands so tightly that he actually complained about it to me post-birth. He spoke words of encouragement as I moaned through the contraction: "It hurts, but you can do it" and "This one's almost over, you're doing great!" This was really helpful mentally.

My husband and doula were both so vital to the process that at one point, my doula had stepped into the curtained-off supply area of the room to pump breast milk for her own infant back at home, and I literally couldn't manage without her for even a few contractions, so she popped back over the curtain, operating a breast pump in one hand and applying pressure to my back with the other. This may have been awkward for her or for my husband who was in clear view now of breast milk leaking from her boob into a bottle, but I sure as hell didn't care. Similarly, I lashed out at my husband who was sending a text to family to tell them it was getting close to the time they should head to the hospital. I needed him right there with me to hold on to during the contraction.

Like many natural birthing mamas, I began to doubt myself and my ability to continue. When this happens, it means that birth is imminent. Some women say ridiculous statements during this time, like "Let's go home and have this baby later." I was less outlandish, although this was pretty unexpected for me, and simply said, as with my first, that I changed my mind and wanted an epidural. My husband honored my original and adamant wishes and told me no, that I didn't need it. If he had wavered instead, I'm sure that nurse would have had the anesthesiologist in my room in a jiffy just to prove me wrong. I'd like to think that I wouldn't have gone through with it, but I'll never know because he didn't give me the chance, and for that I am grateful to him.

At about 1:30 a.m., just five hours after the start of Pitocin, I started to feel the urge to push. I hadn't felt this with Dylan's birth, maybe because he was so small, but when I felt it this time, it was unmistakable, so I knew it really must be the end. Again, my midwife came to check me, and I was about 9 or more centimeters, thank goodness, so she was able to manually move the remaining cervix to get me to 10.

I first pushed sitting on my knees facing the back of the bed, as I had with my son. Then I thought it would be helpful to see what was going on more, so I turned around sitting upright, and they brought in the mirror so I could watch.

With each contraction, someone was holding up each of my legs. My doula told me to make a "C" with my body while pushing. She reminded me to "push with my bottom, not with my face" if she saw that I was tensing my face during a push. I watched myself slowly open, and remembered how the slowness of it had been discouraging with Dylan. That's how it's supposed to happen, I reminded myself. And in no time at all (well, 20 minutes in real time), I suddenly saw the whole head crowning. The midwife asked my husband if he wanted to make the catch. He quickly put a scrub gown over his clothes and gloves over his hands. She guided him in delivering the head, and helped him pull out the shoulders when I pushed the body out. As the baby emerged, I reached down to receive her and immediately brought her to my chest. Then my husband announced it was a girl. I didn't believe it and made him repeat the news.

I held her for quite a while. The nurse wiped her down and suctioned her while she was in my arms. After about a half hour, the nurse took her to the other side of the room to be weighed.

Again, it wasn't perfect. It didn't go quite as I'd hoped. (I'm convinced there is a button in my uterus that my babies push to make my water break before they have any intention of vacating the place. Maybe it's their first way of letting me know who they think is in charge.) But I took events as they came. I modified my expectations when I needed to, while keeping true to the fundamental principles of my intentions.

Liv Alexandra Rauseo was born at 2:07 a.m. on April 28, 2011.

Fiona Mallory, born April 11, 2014

For most people, being 38 weeks pregnant is the beginning of the end. But for me, it seemed like a pregnant eternity. I had been waiting for labor to begin since about 35 weeks. After my first baby came at 34 weeks and my second at 37, I never imagined I could go much further than that. So when my 38-week appointment rolled around, I asked the midwife, "What do we do at a 38-week visit, anyway?"

I had been experiencing Braxton Hicks and also real contractions on and off since about 36 and a half weeks. Each and every time I felt that tightening in my belly, I assumed I was in labor. For me, "labor" had always started, not with actual labor, but with my water spontaneously breaking, followed by no labor at all for two days. So I didn't really know how to recognize any other early signs of labor.

When I experienced pretty steady Braxton Hicks on Thursday afternoon for several hours at 38 weeks and 2 days pregnant, I thought this might be it. And of course, it still might not be. "I just wish I could get a clear sign so I would know for sure," I said aloud to my husband. I was not really sick of being pregnant, just very curious how much longer it would last and a little anxious about not knowing. Less than five minutes later, I felt a slight wetness in my pajama pants, and I casually went to the bathroom to evaluate the situation. I told David my water may have just broken, but I don't think he really believed me after the last week and a half full of false "I think I might be in labor" warnings. It wasn't until several minutes later when a huge gush came out of me, soaking through my maxi pad, pajama pants and onto my bedroom carpet, that I completely believed myself. Indeed, I was in labor!

It was 9 p.m. on April 10. I texted my doula, Heather, and my birth photographer, Danna. I called the hospital and spoke to Mary, the midwife working the night shift. She said to come in within 12 to 24 hours. I said I was sure I'd be in touch sooner. For the next couple hours, my contractions were mild but steady. I timed them using the contraction app I had downloaded three years earlier for Liv's birth but never used since I'd ended up being induced with her.

At 11 p.m. I told Danna she should probably head over. She was coming from 40 minutes away and I was nervous my labor could pick up speed quickly at any point. By the time she arrived at midnight, my contractions, previously five minutes apart, had fallen to 10 or 15 minutes apart. I told her to get some rest in my guest room and that I'd wake her when they picked up again. David got some rest too, and I sort of slept in between contractions, still timing them with the app. When I saw they were more regular again, maybe five to seven minutes apart and lasting a minute each around 3 a.m., I told Heather to come, and I woke Danna up.

Heather arrived at 4 a.m. We had a little labor party in my bedroom: David sitting on the floor, me in child's pose practicing my Ojai breath during every contraction while Heather rubbed my back; Danna shooting pictures of my dog, Lucy, looking at me like I was nuts.

In between, things were totally calm. We had conversations that stopped and started with my contractions. We talked about when to go to the hospital. Heather seemed to think I was good to stay at home for a while longer, wanting to make sure an early arrival to the hospital wouldn't take my birth plan off track. We also had some logistics involved in the timing – beginning at 6 a.m., my big kids could start to wake up, and my in-laws had to come over to watch them. My niece was going to be dropped off at my house around 7 a.m. to be babysat by my in-laws as well. I wanted to bypass all of this commotion, so we decided we would head for the hospital just before 6.

I wasn't sure how much longer this would take and I knew I wouldn't be allowed to eat once I arrived, so I thought it was a good idea to have a snack. David brought up plates of bagels and cream cheese and we all had breakfast in my bed.

Prior to leaving the house, I was still able to speak between contractions. As soon as I ate a few bites of my bagel and got up to make an exit, the game quickly changed. I was struggling the whole 10-minute car ride. I texted my mom and my sisters to give them an update and ballpark of when to arrive to the hospital. Normally an avid texter, I was in no state for digital banter, and left my sister (who was also pregnant) hanging when she asked for a selfie-video of me in labor so she could see what it was like. As we walked into the ER entrance (since the main entrance hadn't yet opened), I told David if I wasn't yet in transition (8 centimeters) to please kill me.

Heather pushed my wheelchair from the ER to L&D while David carried our bags, and Danna captured the whole thing. Janitors watched as we stopped several times during that short walk so I could stand up and brace myself for each contraction.

When we finally got to triage at about 6 a.m., they wouldn't let my whole entourage in the small room, so just David and I went in. The triage lady asked me ridiculously unimportant questions like when my last menstrual cycle was (ummm, 9 months ago) and if I had an advance directive and whether or not I'd brought it with me (how about you just don't kill me while I'm here). We paused filling out her questionnaire while I experienced contractions and held onto David in excruciating pain.

The midwife, Mary, came in and did a cervical exam. She said I was 6-7 centimeters dilated, which was not as far along as I'd hoped, but I decided to live anyway. Heather reminded me it was just a number. To be honest, I didn't really have time to be that discouraged.

We were quickly moved to a labor and delivery room – the one with a birthing tub that had just been installed two months earlier – and I asked them to fill it up immediately. I was told I had to be put on the monitor for 30 minutes first, per hospital protocol. Once the nurse placed two belts around my belly, I had the distinct urge to relieve my bowels. I whined like a 3-year-old to please let me go to the bathroom. With the belts still Velcroed around me, I hobbled over to the toilet, where, of course, despite the enormous rectal pressure, I didn't really have to poop.

Once I returned to the bed, I said there was no way I could lie down through another contraction, so they raised the bed up allowing me to lean on it from a standing position. I begged them to let me get in the tub, to make an exception with regard to the monitoring rule, but Mary said I had to continue. I silently cursed myself for not coming to the hospital sooner so that I'd have been in better shape during this required monitoring period.

Mary asked me if I intended to give birth in the tub and then told me something about how the American College of Obstetricians and Gynecologists, the American Academy of Pediatrics or some other important organization has deemed water birth "experimental," and did I still want to proceed given that information.

Somehow I got through the monitoring period, during which a nurse inserted an IV lock in my right hand, stopping the process every 20 seconds while I had another contraction and I squeezed her gloved fingers as hard as I could. I had previously been squeezing David's hands, but I guess at that point I grabbed whatever was within reach. My eyes were mostly closed throughout this time and I had little idea of anything going on around me. All I could hear were my extremely loud moans through every contraction. I thought to myself that the whole hospital surely could hear me. I tried to remember to use deep sounds instead of shrieky ones but I can't promise which kind came out. Someone else must have reminded me as well, and said "You're going to lose your voice," and I did, in fact, have a hoarse voice after the birth.

I was elated when Mary gave me the green light to get in the tub. Heather tied on my bikini top and I climbed into the warm water. I felt some relief upon immersion but not the complete absence of pain I'd heard or read about from other women who have labored in water. I leaned forward during each contraction, and felt a need to push, even though I assumed I was still only about 7 centimeters dilated. Unlike my other births, I never thought about or asked for an epidural. Somehow, it wasn't an option to even mention it this time. Instead, I kept thinking a couple hours into the future. I envisioned myself in the mother-baby room where I'd be snuggling with a brand new, dark-haired little newborn, this tremendous pain a vague memory. I couldn't wait for that reality. When I voiced that I couldn't do it anymore – I actually said I wanted to go home at one point – Heather reminded me that I was just bringing my baby down, and I tried hard to keep focus on my vision.

After a little while on my own in the tub, I asked David to join me. I questioned him several times on whether he'd texted our families first to make sure they were on their way. I heard some soft chuckles from hospital staff that I was concerning myself with this at that exact moment.

I rested my weight on David's chest and began using controlled pushes during each contraction. I wasn't necessarily pushing to get the baby out; I was just attempting to relieve the enormous pressure. I was almost pushing and sucking in at the same time, afraid to give in to the process completely. At some point, Mary checked me again and said I was fully dilated and to push as I please. I asked for a mirror, which was wheeled in and positioned so I could see my progress.

For a little while, it looked like a whole lot of nothing happening. And then, the pressure sensation changed somewhat, and I could literally feel the head moving through my pelvis. "It's coming!" I shouted, and I knew I was really close. I pushed with an intense desire to finish the job and I felt the ring of fire as the head began to emerge. While the baby was crowning, I got a break from contractions, and I just hung out for a little while with a head about a quarter of the way out of my vagina. I begged aloud to no one in particular for another contraction to come so I could give another push. When one finally came and I delivered the head, I felt a sweet relief, which was only paralleled a couple pushes later when the body followed. I reached down and brought the baby to me. I had to look for what seemed like a couple minutes to confirm the gender as David's arm was in the way. And then I saw I'd been carrying my precious baby girl.

Fiona Mallory, my very last baby, was born on April 11, 2014 at 7:10 a.m. in the water. I consider her entrance to the world to have been my ideal natural-birth-at-the-hospital experience.

Acknowledgements

It only took me about nine months to create each of my children, while this book took me nearly two years. It's no wonder I feel like I've given birth yet again (naturally, of course).

First, I have to thank my husband, David, for introducing me to the idea of natural birth. I would be a very different person today if you hadn't had the *chutzpah* to tell your pregnant wife how she should deliver her child. Also, I thank you for suggesting I write this book. I'm sure you were just sick of me talking about it all the time, and you thought this would be a good outlet for my enthusiasm, but nonetheless, thank you.

Next I want to thank my personal birth people. Along with David, these ladies were instrumental to me achieving the natural births of my children.

Elena Varipatis Baker of EVB Doula Services – I wouldn't have dreamed of having a baby without you there (that is, of course, until you decided to move out of state right after I became pregnant with number three!). You have a gift for providing unparalleled birth support to laboring mothers, and it impresses me.

Heather Brown of Yoga Birth Baltimore (yogabirthbaltimore.org) – your husband put the natural birth bug in my husband's ear that started me on the road to here, and I thank you for lending us *The Business of Being Born*. You have played so many roles during my pregnancies: childbirth educator, yoga instructor, doula, and friend. Your work in the local birth community is an inspiration to me.

Danna Stumberg of Stumberg Photography (stumbergphotography.com) – you captured the most beautiful images of one of the most important days of my life. You are truly talented beyond any words I can think of to describe the gift you have. My only regret was that I didn't know you for my first two births!

Paula McCabe, CNM, who attended my son's birth. You also happened to be working a couple of shifts while I was attempting to go into labor at home with my second child. Your advice for natural induction, your permission to wait before going to the hospital, and your personal story of surviving Pitocin without an epidural were all greatly appreciated.

Monique Klapka, CNM, who attended my first daughter's birth. You also happened to be working when I met with the high-risk OB while waiting for labor with my son, and you were the one who told me I didn't have to be induced as she proposed. I liked you before this conversation, but after, I knew without a doubt that you were my advocate, and I thank you.

Gigi Moore, CNM, who worked with me during my last pregnancy (and the many neuroses that seemed to accompany it!). You showed much support of my birth choices over many months and I'm thankful. I wish I could keep seeing you regularly, but not quite enough to have another baby!

Mary Knauer, CNM, who attended my newest baby's water birth. Your peaceful demeanor and hands-off approach were contributing factors to what I consider my perfect birth experience.

And all the pregnant women and new moms I met with and talked to on the phone and over email: You shared with me your time, thoughts, plans, fears, and experiences when this book was still gestating and I didn't quite know where it was going. Many of you gave me much-needed words of encouragement, too. Thank you to: Alissa DeBernardo, Emily Engelman, Amanda Favreau, Lauren Heslep, Kate Hummel, Emily Lancaster, Anne (last name omitted), Laurie Mazelin, Sarah Nguyen, Monica Pascatore, Rita Piel, Rachel Rossbach, Shannon Snow, Rebecca Teaff, Sarrah Yoder and Christie Zimmerman. The quotes at the beginning of each chapter come from some of these moms who birthed their babies, each in her own way.

To my first readers: I thank you for your time, your honesty, and your awesome suggestions. This is a much better book because of you. Thank you to: Amy Brendler, Jamie Ollins, Christie Zimmerman, Elena Varipatis Baker, Jessie Stadd, Heather Brown, Jane Kaufman and Monique Klapka, CNM.

And finally, to my children. Dylan and Liv, if you guys weren't around, well, let's be honest, I could have written this book much faster, but then I wouldn't have had anything to say at all. Fiona, I wrote this book before you were even here, but your entrance into the world fulfilled my hopes and dreams for what I longed for in a natural birth experience. My happiest moments were the first time I held each of you in my arms, though every time I've hugged you since then has been pretty amazing, too.

Follow the author at www.facebook.com/MainstreamMama

Made in the USA
Lexington, KY
30 June 2015